A-Z Notes in Radiological Practice and Reporting

Series Editors
Carlo Nicola De Cecco
Andrea Laghi

Pasquale Paolantonio
Clarisse Dromain

Imaging of Small Bowel, Colon and Rectum

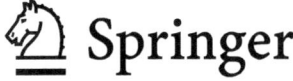 Springer

Pasquale Paolantonio
Department of Radiology
San Giovanni Hospital
Roma
Italy

Clarisse Dromain
Department of Radiology
Institut de Cancerologie Gustav
Roussy
VilleJuif - Paris
France

ISBN 978-88-470-5488-2   ISBN 978-88-470-5489-9   (eBook)
DOI 10.1007/978-88-470-5489-9
Springer Milan Heidelberg New York Dordrecht London

Printed on acid-free paper

Springer is part of Springer Science+Business Media (www.springer.com)

Foreword to this Series

A-Z Notes in Radiological Practice and Reporting is a new series of practical guides dedicated to residents and general radiologists. The series was born, thanks to the original idea to bring to the public attention a series of notes, collected by doctors and fellows during their clinical activity and attendance at international academic institutions. Those brief notes were critically reviewed, sometimes integrated, cleaned up, and organized in the form of an A–Z glossary, to be usable by a third reader.

The ease and speed of consultation and the agility in reading were behind the construction of this series and were the reasons why the booklets are organized alphabetically, primarily according to disease or condition. The number of illustrations has been deliberately reduced and focused only on those ones relevant to the specific entry.

Residents and general radiologists will find in these booklets numerous quick answers to frequent questions occurring during radiological practice, which will be useful in daily activity for planning exams and radiologic reporting.

Each single entry typically includes a short description of pathological and clinical characteristics, guidance on selection of the most appropriate imaging technique, a schematic review of potential diagnostic clues, and useful tips and tricks.

The series will include the most relevant topics in radiology, starting with cardiac imaging and continuing with the gastrointestinal tract, liver, pancreas and bile ducts, and genitourinary apparatus during the first 2 years. More arguments will be covered in the next issues.

The Editors put a lot of their efforts in selecting the most appropriate colleagues willing to exchange with readers their own experiences in their respective fields. The result is a combination of experienced professors, enthusiastic researchers, and young talented radiologists working together within a single framework project, with the primary aim of making their knowledge available for residents and general practitioners.

We really do hope that this series can meet the satisfaction of the readers and can help them in their daily radiological practice.

Latina, Italy   Andrea Laghi
                                                              Carlo Nicola De Cecco

Contents

A

Abdominal Angina

- Abdominal angina or *chronic mesenteric ischemia* is a form of intermittent mesenteric ischemia in severe arterial stenosis with inadequate bowel perfusion triggered by food ingestion.
- Postprandial pain when blood flow goes away from the intestine due to the so-called gastric steal. Patients present typically with weight loss and clinical signs of malabsorption.
- Duplex US can depict celiac trunk occlusion; a peak systolic velocity >160 cm/s in the celiac trunk during fasting has an SE of 57 % and SP of 100 % for 50 % stenosis.
- CT enterography (or CT enteroclysis) is a powerful diagnostic tool in the identification of both splanchnic vessel strictures and bowel wall changes.
- Biphasic scan is required in CT enterography by acquiring and arterial phase scan similar to CTA (CT angiography) and a delayed scan (enteric phase). CT enterography owing to contrast medium injection similar to *CTA* (*CT angiography*) with accurate post-processing (MIP, MPR, 3D VR) can easily

P. Paolantonio, C. Dromain, *Imaging of Small Bowel, Colon and Rectum*,
A-Z Notes in Radiological Practice and Reporting,
DOI 10.1007/978-88-470-5489-9_1, © Springer-Verlag Italia 2014

depict with high accuracy strictures of the celiac trunk, SMA, and IMA showing also peripheric splanchnic vessels while the "enteric phase" (70 s after contrast medium injection) allows optimal evaluation of bowel wall changes.

- CT enterography is able to depict chronic ischemic bowel wall changes in patients with abdominal angina such as bowel wall thinning, mucosal fold flattening, and long and smooth bowel strictures. Diagnostic information similar to those of CT enterography can be reached also using *MR enterography* or *MR enteroclysis*.

Abdominopelvic Incoordination

- Abdominopelvic incoordination (pelvic floor incoordination) is a condition characterized by impaired coordination between pelvic floor (e.g., puborectal muscle) relaxation and abdominal wall motion leading to chronic constipation and obstructed defecation syndrome.
- MR defecography is a valid tool to diagnose the abdominopelvic incoordination and to differentiate it from other possible causes of *obstructed defecation* syndrome such as descending perineum, rectal prolapse, and rectocele. This differential diagnosis is essential in treatment planning of obstructed defecation. In case of abdominopelvic incoordination, the clue sign at MR defecography is represented by paradox contraction of the puborectal muscle during defecation with missing anorectal angle opening leading to impaired evacuation.

"Accordion" Sign

- Accordion sign is a pattern of large bowel wall thickening suggesting acute inflammatory changes (acute infective colitis or pseudomembranous colitis). Marked thickening of haustral

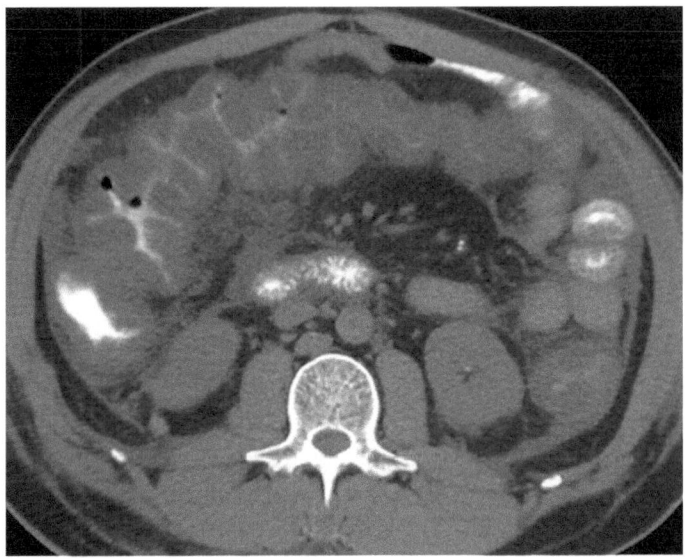

Fig. 1 The marked and diffuse colonic fold thickening at the level of the transverse colon in this patient suffering from pseudomembranous colitis mimics an accordion appearance. This finding represents the so-called accordion sign: a sign of acute inflammatory colonic wall changes

fold due to submucosa edema mimics an accordion appearance (Fig. 1).

Acute Mesenteric Ischemia

- Etiology of acute mesenteric ischemia is represented by reduced blood flow to the bowel through mesenteric vessels due to *occlusive embolus* (*occlusive mesenteric infarction*) or SMA thrombosis or due to systemic low flow (hypovolemia, cardiac failure, intraoperative hypotension) in preexisting atherosclerosis of SMA (*nonocclusive mesenteric ischemia*).

- Acute mesenteric ischemia may be present also in case of *venous thrombosis* (SMV, IMV, or portal vein) or may complicate bowel obstruction in case of *strangulation* by adhesion, volvulus, incarcerated hernia, or intussusception. Finally acute intestinal ischemia may be the manifestation of intestinal *vasculitis* or inflammatory abdominal process such as pancreatitis or peritonitis.

- In case of occlusive mesenteric ischemia, usually occlusion is due to an embolus at the level of SMA bifurcation; if the embolus is located distal to the middle colic artery, no compensatory collateral vessel is available leading to mesenteric infarction.

- Increased WBC is a common finding in case of acute mesenteric ischemia. Abdominal pain and gross rectal bleeding represent symptoms. Ischemia may involve any tract of the small bowel; concerning the colon, the distal transverse colon and cecum are the most common location. Consequence of acute mesenteric ischemia is represented by transmural infarction with perforation in case of irreversible ischemia or by restitution of bowel wall due to collaterals with fibrosis of the bowel with possible stricture formation.

- Contrast-enhanced CT of the abdomen represents the imaging test of choice. Unenhanced CT scan followed by CTA of splanchnic vessels with dedicated post-processing acquiring also a delayed "enteric" CT phase (70 s) represents the winning CT protocol. Using such protocol detailed vascular information as well as direct assessment of bowel wall ischemic changes are easily detected.

- Ischemic bowel wall changes are represented by bowel wall thickening with target appearance (alternating layers of high and low attenuation). In case of severe ischemia, reduced bowel wall enhancement is expected as well as wall thinning. The bowel wall usually is dilated and distended by fluid. Increased wall enhancement and delayed enhancement are possible due to venous congestion secondary to stasis. Intestinal pneumatosis is a sign of irreversible disease.

Adenomatous Polyp

- An adenomatous polyp is a benign neoplastic growth with variable malignant potential, representing proliferation of glandular epithelium in the lumen of the colon–rectum. Several histopathology subtypes are described: the tubular, tubulovillous, villous, and sessile serrated. Malignant potential is associated with the degree of dysplasia, the histopathological subtype of polyp (5 % risk of cancer for tubular, 20 % for tubulovillous, and 40 % for villous), and the size of polyp (from <1 % for polyp <1 cm to 15 % for polyp ≥2 cm).

  Although most adenomatous polyp is sporadic, it also is lined to some inherited disorders including the familial adenomatous polyposis, the Gardner syndrome, and the Lynch syndrome (HNPCC).
- There are usually no symptoms. When present, symptoms may include rectal bleeding and bloody stools.
- Screening plays an important role to prevent the transformation of polyp into cancer. People over age 50 should consider having screening test. Screening tests are represented by fecal occult blood test (FOBT), optical colonoscopy (that allows polypectomy), and *virtual colonoscopy*. People with a family history of colon cancer or colon polyps may need to be screened by colonoscopy at an earlier age (40 years).
- When a polyp has been removed, follow-up colonoscopy is usually recommended 1–10 years later, depending on the age, the number of polyps depicted on the previous colonoscopy, and the size and pathology subtype; usually a 5-year follow-up is recommended.

Adenomatous Polyposis, Familial

- Familial adenomatous polyposis (FAP) is an inherited condition resulting more often from mutations in the APC gene (autosomal dominant), less frequently from mutations in the MUTYH gene (autosomal recessive) that predispose to colorectal cancers. Hundreds or thousands of premalignant adenomatous colonic polyps appear around the age of 16 years old (from 7 to 36). Unless the colon is removed, these polyps will become malignant and most of patients will develop colon cancer by the age of 40. Less severe form, called attenuated familial adenomatous polyposis, is characterized with a lower number of polyp (mean 30), a location of polyps predominant in the proximal colon, and an average age of colorectal cancer of 55 years.
- Extracolic signs may also suggest the diagnosis of FAP: pigmented lesions of the retina, jaw cysts, sebaceous cysts, and osteoma. The combination of FAP, osteomas of the skull, thyroid cancer, fibromas, and epidermoid cysts as well as the occurrence of desmoid tumors in approximately 15 % is termed Gardner syndrome. The combination of FAP with brain tumors, glioblastomas, astrocytomas, or medulloblastomas is termed Turcot syndrome.

Adhesive Intestinal Band

- Adhesive intestinal band is a band of scar tissue in the abdominal cavity binding the intestinal loop one with each other or to other abdominal organ or to the abdominal wall. Adhesive band may be thin sheets or thick fibrous band.
- Intestinal adhesion is a common complication of abdominopelvic surgery; however, they can develop also in patients that

never had surgery as a repairing mechanism of abdominal tissue due to different injuries such as infection, trauma, or radiation. Most adhesions are painless and do not cause complications. However, adhesions cause the majority of small bowel obstructions in adults and are believed to contribute to the development of chronic pelvic pain.

- At CT scan, it is difficult to visualize the adhesive band itself; however, in case of adhesive causing intestinal obstruction, the so-called fat notch sign visible at the level of the transitional zone can identify directly the adhesive band causing intestinal obstruction.
- In the pelvic district in women with chronic pelvic pain, MRI is a useful tool to visualize adhesive band between the small bowel, sigmoid colon, uterus, and adnexa; in such patients the adhesive bands are thick fibrotic bands developing in the course of endometriosis, and therefore MRI can visualize low-signal-intensity tissue on T2-weighted images (fibrotic tissue) as well as high-signal-intensity foci on T1-weighted images due to the presence of hemoglobin degradation product.

Adynamic Ileus

- Adynamic ileus (paralytic ileus, nonobstructive ileus) is represented by the inability to push fluid along the bowel lumen due to a derangement or impaired proper peristaltic distal propulsion of intestinal content without a mechanical intestinal obstruction.
- Possible causes of adynamic ileus are represented by the following: postoperative ileus (usually resolves by 4th postoperative day), visceral pain (ureteral stone, common bile duct stone, twisted ovarian cyst, blunt abdominal or chest trauma), intra-abdominal inflammation or infection (peritonitis,

appendicitis, cholecystitis, pancreatitis, salpingitis, abdominal abscess, gastroenteritis), ischemic bowel disease, anticholinergic drug assumption, neuromuscular disorder (diabetes, hypothyroidism, porphyries, uremia, hypokalemia, paraplegia), retroperitoneal disease (hemorrhage, abscess), chest disease (lower lobe pneumonia, pleuritis, myocardial infarction, pericarditis), and systemic disease (septic shock). X-ray abdominal plain film can easily identify multiple air–liquid levels involving both the large and small bowel.

- CT scan is essential for differential diagnosis between obstructive and nonobstructive ileus and for the identification of the origin of adynamic ileus. If Gastrografin ® is administered orally, a delayed but free passage of contrast material is expected in case of adynamic ileus despite the obstructive ileus; X-ray plain film can be easily performed to monitor the passage of contrast material over time.

- Adynamic ileus may also involve an isolated loop of the small or large bowel (sentinel loop) due to the presence of an adjacent acute inflammatory process (pancreatitis, cholecystitis, appendicitis, diverticulitis, or acute ureteral colic).

Angiodysplasia of the Colon

- Angiodysplasia is an arteriovenous malformation in the bowel submucosa. It is more frequently localized in the cecum and in the ascending colon and less frequently in the left colon.

- It is responsible of chronic low-grade intermittent bleeding and, occasionally, of massive bleeding.

- Identification of angiodysplasia at cross-sectional imaging is challenging. However acquiring an arterial CT phase and performing MPR reconstruction and/or MIP reconstruction, a cluster of arterial vessels along the antimesenteric border may be the unique sign of angiodysplasia. Intraluminal blush of contrast material due to active bleeding is quite unusual. *Video capsule endoscopy* is recommended in a patient with GI bleeding with negative result of endoscopic studies and CT studies in a patient without intestinal strictures.

Anisakiasis

- Anisakiasis is a parasitic disease of the GI tract due to the ingestion of Anisakis larvae present in raw fish.
- The site of penetration of larvae determines the clinical form (gastric anisakiasis, intestinal anisakiasis). Gastric anisakiasis symptoms are represented by acute gastric pain and vomiting few hours after ingestion; eosinophilia is common.
- Intestinal anisakiasis presents with diffuse abdominal tenderness, vomiting, and abdominal pain. Imaging features are aspecific showing diffuse small bowel wall thickening due to marked edema and eosinophilic infiltrates leading to irregular nominal narrowing; ascites is commonly associated and lab test shows commonly leukocytosis. If eosinophilia is present it may help in suggesting diagnosis of parasitic infection. Colon anisakiasis is rare and the differential diagnosis is with colon carcinoma.

Anorectal Angle

- The anorectal angle (ARA) is formed by longitudinal axis of the rectum with the longitudinal axis of the anal canal at the anorectal junction (Fig. 2). ARA is one of the most important contributions to anal continence, and its normal

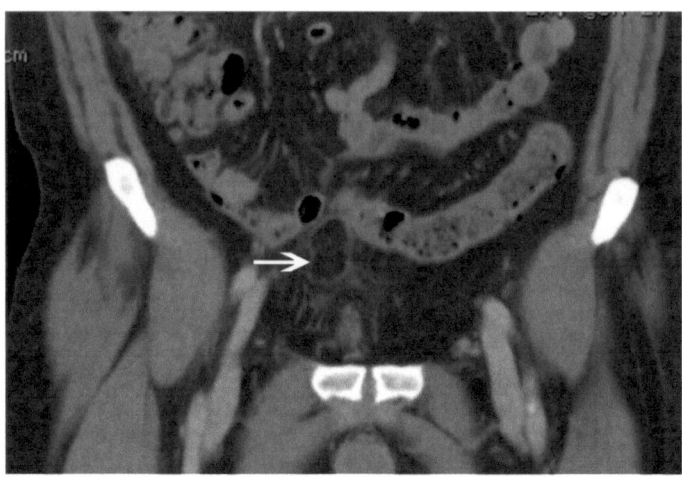

Fig. 2 Image shows a coronal MPR reconstruction of a CT scan in a patient with epiploic appendagitis. An oval fat-density mass (*arrow*) with surrounding fat stranding is visible adjacent to the colon

value at rest is 90°. Anorectal angle opening up to 180° during defecation is due to relaxation of the puborectal muscle. In some cases of obstructed defecation, the puborectal muscle contraction during defecation leads to the so-called abdominopelvic incoordination (Fig. 3).

Anti-TNF Alpha (Infliximab®)

• Anti-TNF alpha is a chimeric human anti-TNF alpha antibody approved by FDA for biologic treatment of several autoimmune disease comprising Crohn's disease. This antibody

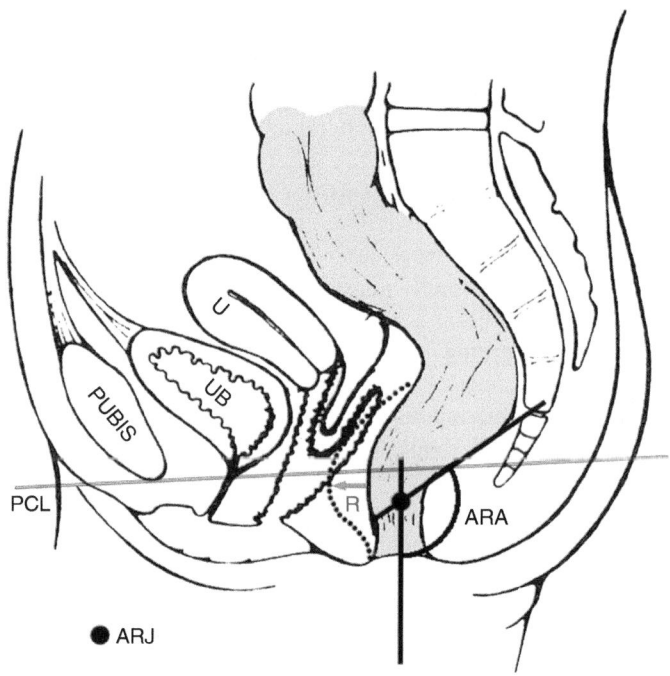

Fig. 3 The graphic illustrates the anorectal angle (*ARA*). *PCL* represent the pubococcygeal line; *ARJ* represents the anorectal junction. *R* indicates the anterior rectal wall, and the *gray arrow* shows the direction of anterior rectal wall bulging and rectocele formation

allows a downregulation of the immune system leading to reduction of inflammatory activity in Crohn's disease patients and healing of fistula in Crohn's disease. However a patient candidate to biologic therapy should be carefully selected since this therapy may have several adverse reactions (activation of infective disease due to downregulation of immune system).

Aortomesenteric Compression Syndrome

- Aortomesenteric compression syndrome (also known as aortomesenteric nutcracker syndrome) is a rare condition caused by extrinsic compression of the horizontal portion of the duodenum by means of the superior mesenteric artery due to a thinning of the adipose tissue between the abdominal aorta and superior mesenteric artery.
- Symptoms are usually nonspecific and intermittent; the most common symptom is represented by postprandial epigastric pain and vomiting.
- Diagnosis is made by means of CTA of the abdominal aorta. If the aortomesenteric compression syndrome is clinically suspected, CTA should be performed after patient oral water overload that allows a better definition of the extrinsic substenosis of the duodenum. In young patients, MRA of the abdominal aorta should be preferred than CTA in order to avoid patient exposure to ionizing radiation.

Appendagitis, Epiploic

- Epiploic appendagitis is a rare inflammation of one of the 100 epiploic appendages of the colon due to torsion, venous thrombosis of the appendages itself, or inflammation coming from adjacent organ (appendicitis, diverticulitis). Epiploic appendagitis usually has a spontaneous resolution, and therefore treatment is conservative and surgery is not recommended.
- The patient presents with abrupt onset of localized abdominal pain (more often in the right lower quadrant) gradually resolving in 3–7 days.

- At US a solid hyperechoic ovoid mass near the colon can be appreciated.
- CT is the most sensitive test showing pericolic oval-shaped pedunculated mass (1–4 cm) with fat attenuation (−60 HU) with fat stranding like a focal pericolic mass-forming fat stranding. The differential diagnosis of such findings is with greater omentum infarction.

Appendicitis

- Appendicitis is represented by inflammation of the cecal appendix wall due to obstruction of appendiceal lumen by lymphoid hyperplasia, fecalith, or, less commonly, cecal Crohn's disease or cecal tumor (in adult/old population).
- The continued production of mucus in case on obstructed appendiceal lumen leads to increased intraluminal pressure with lumen distension and venous engorgement followed by arterial compromise evolving in tissue ischemia when intraluminal pressure exceeds capillary perfusion pressure. Necrotic changes and perforation are common complications of untreated acute appendicitis leading to abscess or phlegmon formation in the right iliac fossa with localized or diffuse peritonitis.
- Acute appendicitis represents 1–4 % of all acute abdominal pain in children, and the peak age is within the second decade; thereafter incidence declines.
- Pain is mild and poorly localized in the epigastrium and periumbilical area for 4–6 h then tends to migrate to the RLQ with McBurney signs (72 %) and becomes continuous and

more severe, accompanied by nausea, vomiting, and low-grade fever. Perforation is suspected if temperature is >38 °C with leukocytosis and shift of WBC count to the left. Despite the clinical findings, appendicitis diagnosis may be uncertain in 20–35 % of cases in elderly patients, ovulating women, infants, or young children.

- Graded compression US using both low-frequency convex and high-frequency linear probe has good results (85 % SE, 92 % SP, 78–96 % accuracy). Appendix is visualized at US as a noncompressible, blind-ending tubular aperistaltic structure just in 2 % of normal adults but in 50 % of normal children. A laminated appendiceal wall with target appearance (>6 mm in total diameter) and mural wall >2 mm is a very specific sign of appendicitis (81 % SP). Other signs are represented by fluid lumen distension, pericecal fluid, and increased periappendiceal echogenicity. False-negative US causes are represented by inability to adequate compression of the right iliac fossa, aberrant location of the appendix (retrocecal), and appendiceal perforation, while false-positive US causes are represented by normal appendix mistaken for appendicitis or alternative diagnosis (Crohn's disease, inflammatory pelvic disease, inflamed Meckel diverticulum).

- CT has 87–100 % SE, 89–98 % SP, and 92–98 % accuracy with NPV ranging from 95 to 100 %. Normal appendix is visualized in 67–100 % of subjects. Abnormal appendix has the following CT signs: distended lumen (diameter >7 mm), circumferential wall thickening, target appearance after CM injection, visualization of appendicolith, periappendicular inflammation with fat stranding, local fascial thickening, and free peritoneal fluid.

- Perforations of appendix CT sign are represented by nonvisualization of the appendix (fragmentation) with pericecal abscess (poorly encapsulated fluid collection ± extraluminal air) or phlegmon (pericecal soft tissue mass).

- MRI has a limited role in diagnosing acute appendicitis; it is suggested in selected cases when clinical findings and US are equivocal in pregnant patients.

Apple Core Lesion

- An apple core lesion is an imaging feature due to a mass that narrows or encircles a tubular structure. It takes its name from the shape into which the bowel is compressed. It is most often observed in case of stenosing lesion of the colon invading the full thickness of the wall or less frequently the small bowel or the esophagus. This finding is primary described on barium enema examinations and is now currently depicted on CT colonoscopy. Although an apple core lesion is highly suggestive of malignant lesions (adenocarcinoma or lymphoma), it has been described in several diseases including Crohn's disease, chronic ulcerative colitis, ischemic colitis, chlamydia infection, tuberculosis, helminthoma, amebiasis, cytomegalovirus, and villous adenoma and radiosurgery such as high doses of CyberKnife used for treating unresectable abdominal malignancies, for example, pancreatic cancer.

Arcuate Ligament Syndrome

- Arcuate ligament syndrome is a condition characterized by compression of the celiac artery by the median arcuate ligament. The median arcuate ligament is a ligament formed at the base of the diaphragm where the left and right diaphragmatic crura join near the 12th thoracic vertebra. In case of arcuate ligament syndrome, the median arcuate ligament is anterior rather than superior with respect to the celiac trunk resulting in compression of the vessel during patient deep inspiration.

- Diagnosis can be suspected by means of color Doppler US.
- CTA represent the most accurate noninvasive imaging method in the diagnosis of arcuate ligament syndrome by visualizing the extrinsic compression of celiac trunk origin with a hook-shaped contour due to the anomalous insertion of the median arcuate ligament.

Suggested Reading

Amzallag-Bellenger E, Oudjit A, Ruiz A, Cadiot G, Soyer PA, Hoeffel CC (2012) Effectiveness of MR enterography for the assessment of small-bowel diseases beyond Crohn disease. Radiographics 32(5):1423–1444

Boyadzhyan L, Raman SS, Raz S (2008) Role of static and dynamic MR imaging in surgical pelvic floor dysfunction. Radiographics 28(4): 949–967

Brenner H, Chang-Claude J, Rickert A, Seiler CM, Hoffmeister MJ (2012) Risk of colorectal cancer after detection and removal of adenomas at colonoscopy: population-based case–control study. Clin Oncol 30(24):2969–2976

Cademartiri F, Raaijmakers RH, Kuiper JW, van Dijk LC, Pattynama PMT, Krestin GP (2004) Multi–detector row CT angiography in patients with abdominal angina. Radiographics 24(4):969–984

Delabrousse E, Lubrano J, Jehl J, Morati P, Rouget C, Mantion GA, Kastler BA (2009) Small-bowel obstruction from adhesive bands and matted adhesions: CT differentiation. AJR 192:693–697

Graça BM, Freire PA, Brito JB, Ilharco JM, Carvalheiro VM, Caseiro-Alves F (2010) Gastroenterologic and radiologic approach to obscure gastrointestinal bleeding: how, why, and when? Radiographics 30(1):235–252

Horton KM, Corl FM, Fishman EK (2000) CT evaluation of the colon: inflammatory disease. Radiographics 20(2):399–418

Horton KM, Talamini MA, Fishman EK (2005) Median arcuate ligament syndrome: evaluation with CT angiography. Radiographics 25(5): 1177–1182

Kim HC, Yang DM, Jin W, Park SJ (2008) Added diagnostic value of multiplanar reformation of multidetector CT data in patients with suspected appendicitis. Radiographics 28(2):393–405

Paulsen SR, Huprich JE, Fletcher JG, Booya F, Young BM, Fidler JL, Daniel Johnson C, Barlow JM, Franklin Earnest IV (2006) CT enterography as a diagnostic tool in evaluating small bowel disorders: review of clinical experience with over 700 cases. Radiographics 26(3):641–657

Purysko AS, Remer EM, Leão Filho HM, Bittencourt LK, Lima RV, Racy DJ (2011) Beyond appendicitis: common and uncommon gastrointestinal causes of right lower quadrant abdominal pain at multidetector CT. Radiographics 31(4):927–947

Silva AC, Pimenta M, Guimaraes LS (2009) Small bowel obstruction: what to look for. Radiographics 29(2):423–439

B

Backwash Ileitis

- Backwash ileitis is represented by chronic mild inflammatory changes of the terminal ileum due to reflux of cecal material through an incontinent ileocecal valve (spillover phenomenon). Backwash ileitis is commonly associated with ulcerative colitis.

Bascule Cecum

- Bascule cecum (seesaw cecum) is a type of cecal volvulus characterized by the rotation of the cecum anterior to the ascending colon (type I cecal volvulus). Type II cecal volvulus occurs when the distended cecum rotates into the left upper quadrant with an overall "kidney-shaped" cecum.
- Cecal volvulus happens in case of poor fixation of the right colon (10–25 % of population) when the pressure in the colonic lumen increases due to constipation or distal colonic obstruction. Pathophysiology of cecal volvulus

P. Paolantonio, C. Dromain, *Imaging of Small Bowel, Colon and Rectum*,
A-Z Notes in Radiological Practice and Reporting,
DOI 10.1007/978-88-470-5489-9_2, © Springer-Verlag Italia 2014

regards vascular compromise with acute mesenteric torsion with strangulation (arterial and venous obstruction), and luminal distension with increased intraluminal distensions interferes with blood supply leading to perforation.

Beak Sign

- Small bowel beak sign represents a CT sign of small bowel mechanical obstruction indicating the site of obstruction, and it is commonly seen in *closed loop intestinal obstruction*. Small bowel caliber above the obstruction site is dilated, while empty small bowel loop is seen after the site of obstruction. The site of obstruction is referred to the point where intestinal caliber changes from dilated loops to empty loops; this crucial point is known as *transitional zone*. In case of mechanical obstruction due to adhesive band, volvulus, and internal hernia, no solid mass is seen at the transitional zone, and the small bowel just above the transitional zone may show the so-called beak sign.

Behcet Syndrome

- Uncommon chronic multisystem inflammatory disorders characterized by mucocutaneous–ocular symptoms as a triad (aphthous stomatitis, genital ulcers, ocular inflammation). Gut may be involved with intestinal deep penetrating ulcers located at the terminal ileum, cecum, and ascending and transverse colon.
- Differential diagnosis with Crohn's disease and ulcerative colitis is made possible by the integration of clinical, endoscopic, and imaging findings.

Bezoar

- Bezoar is represented by persistent concretions and accumulation in the intestine of foreign matter orally ingested. Bezoar can be composed by poorly digested fibers, seeds of fruits, and/or vegetables (phytobezoar) impacted in the small bowel or by hair (trichobezoar). The site of impaction can be at the level of the stomach, jejunum, or ileum.
- At CT dilated small bowel loops with air–fluid levels are visible above the site of impaction. The bezoar itself is visible and an intraluminal material with fecaloid appearance. Intraluminal fecal material in the small bowel ("small bowel feces sign") can be present also in case of long-standing small bowel obstruction (3–4 days) due to absorption of water of the intraluminal content by bowel mucosa and impaction of ingested fibers above the small bowel strictures. However in case of small bowel feces sign, a clear transitional zone with beak sign or fat notch sign or a mass should be identified at the site of intestinal obstruction.

Bleeding (Gastrointestinal)

- Gastrointestinal bleeding may be related to the upper or lower GI tract with the diving landmark being represented by the Treitz ligament; clinical scenario may suggest the upper or lower origin of GI bleeding.
- Endoscopy represents a crucial test in patients with GI bleeding. However in large group of patients with negative or incomplete endoscopy, imaging plays an important role in patient management. Furthermore endoscopic study of the small bowel is not routinely performed in many centers, while an emerging test is represented by *capsule endoscopy*.

- The imaging test of choice in patients with GI bleeding is represented by CTA of splanchnic vessels. Imaging should be performed when active bleeding is suspected.
- Hyperdense oral contrast medium is contraindicated since intraluminal hyperdense contrast medium may obscure completely the attenuation of intraluminal blood as well as the contrast medium blush during i.v. administration of iodinate contrast medium. Good results are described by using oral hypoattenuating contrast medium (*PEG*, *mannitol solution*, etc.) using a so-called *CT enterography* approach.
- Patients should be scanned with triphasic protocol before i.v. CM administration (to identify intraluminal high density of blood), during arterial phase using bolus-tracking method to optimize timing of arterial phase and during a delayed phase (70 s) to identify intraluminal early or delayed CM blush. Post-processing using MPR, MIP, and 3D VR may be helpful in the identification of bleeding site and causes.

Bochdalek Hernia

- Bochdalek hernia represents from 85 to 90 % of all congenital diaphragmatic hernia; it is caused by posterolateral congenital defect of the diaphragm. Therefore Bochdalek is posterior (80 % right-sided, 15 % left-sided, and 5 % bilateral). Usually Bochdalek hernia is large and presenting in infants opposite to the Morgagni hernia that is usually small showing a central and anterior location and presenting in older children.

Bowel Ischemia

- Bowel ischemia (see also acute mesenteric ischemia) is a reduction of bowel blood supply; it can occur in different clinical scenario (acute or chronic). Etiology of bowel ischemia is represented by a wide spectrum of conditions.
- Major mechanisms of bowel ischemia are represented by arterial occlusion (embolic disease, atheromatous disease, dissecting aortic aneurysm, arteritis) and hypoperfusion (shock, hypovolemia). Other possible etiologies are represented by disseminated intravascular coagulation, direct trauma, antiphospholipid antibody syndrome and radiation exposure (>4,500 cGy), mesenteric venous thrombosis (Fig. 1), or bowel obstruction (strangulation, incarcerated hernia, volvulus, intussusception).
- In case of bowel ischemia, two major clinical scenarios are possible: *acute mesenteric ischemia* (see specific item) or *chronic mesenteric ischemia* (also called abdominal angina). Clinical scenario of chronic mesenteric ischemia is represented by postprandial abdominal pain (due to gastric steal diverting blood flow away from intestine) and weight loss.
- Contrast-enhanced CT is the technique of choice for acute mesenteric ischemia, while for chronic mesenteric ischemia dedicated CT enterography scan protocol is suggested in order to acquire a one-stop-shop examination able to detect vascular abnormalities and bowel wall and lumen chronic changes such as 7–10 cm stricture with upstream dilatation and valvular atrophy.

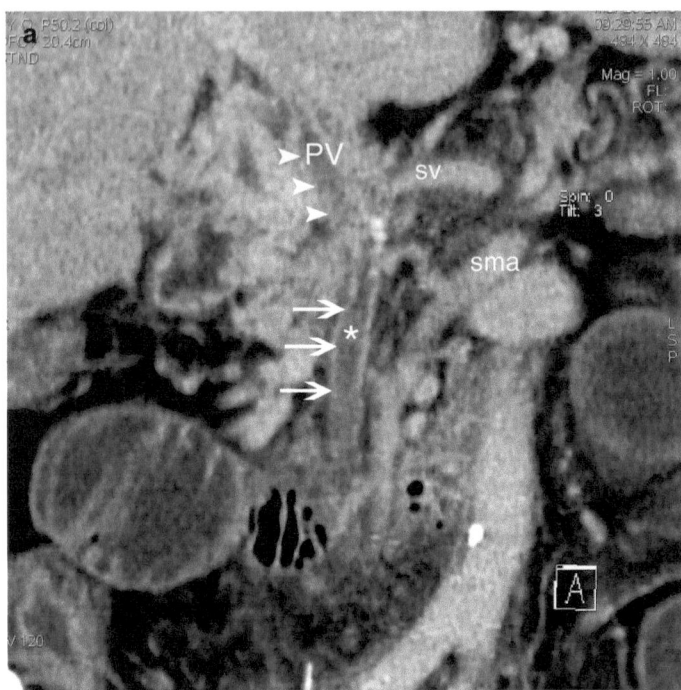

Fig. 1 (**a**) A coronal MPR of a portal-venous-phase contrast-enhanced CT scan is shown. A long filling defect of the portal vein (*arrowheads*) extends into the superior mesenteric vein (*asterisk*) (*arrows*). SMV is also increased in size with fat stranding of mesenteric fat as sign of acute SMV thrombosis. *SV* splenic vein, *SMA* superior mesenteric artery, *PV* portal vein. Portal vein shrinkage with sign of cavernomatous transformation (chronic portal vein thrombosis). The patient presents with acute abdominal pain and leukocytosis. (**b**) Axial image of the same CT study is presented showing diffuse bowel wall thickening of jejunal loops (*J*) as well as the right colon (*C*) with low attenuation of the submucosa and increased density of the mucosa. Free peritoneal fluids are visible as well in the right paracolic space. *Arrowheads* indicate the filling defect into the SMV with mesenteric fat stranding. Overall CT sign refers to acute mesenteric ischemia due to SMV thrombosis

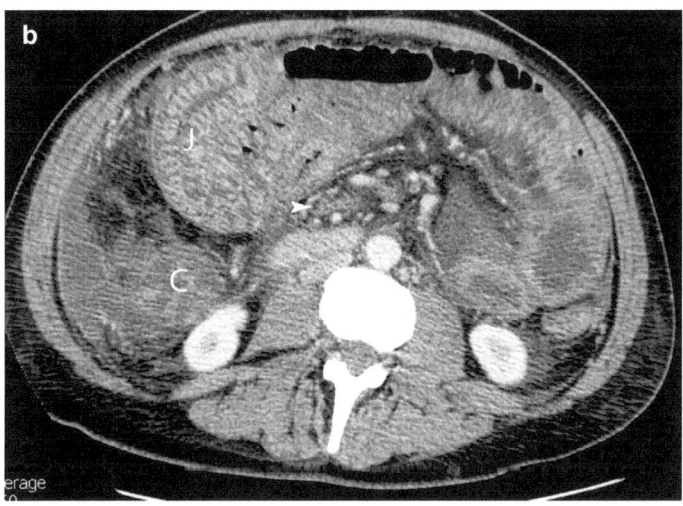

Fig. 1 (continued)

Bowel Obstruction

- Bowel obstruction (*mechanical intestinal obstruction or occlusion*) is a common clinical condition representing about 20 % of all acute abdominal admissions. In 80 % of cases the site of obstruction is located in the small bowel, in 20 % in the colon.
- Three different scenarios are possible: *small bowel obstruction (SBO), small bowel strangulated obstruction, and colonic obstruction.*

Small Bowel Obstruction

- Possible causes of small bowel obstruction can be categorized into *congenital, extrinsic bowel lesion, intrinsic bowel
  lesion, and luminal occlusion.*
- *Congenital* etiology (intestinal atresia, enteric duplication,
  midgut volvulus, mesenteric cyst, Meckel diverticulum) is
  obviously typical in newborn and children.
- *Extrinsic bowel lesion* (most common cause in adults of
  small bowel obstruction) is represented by:

  - Adhesion (50–75 %) from previous surgery or peritonitis
  - Hernia (10 %)
  - Volvulus
  - Extrinsic masses: neoplasm (peritoneal carcinomatosis),
    abscesses, aneurysm, hematoma, and endometriosis

- *Intestinal luminal occlusion* may happen in case of intestinal
  bezoar, gallstone, and intussusception.
- *Intrinsic bowel lesion* leading to bowel occlusion is represented by:

  - Small bowel neoplasm (adenocarcinoma, carcinoid tumor,
    lymphoma, GIST)
  - Inflammatory lesion (Crohn's disease, eosinophilic enteri-
    tis, infection)
  - Vascular lesions (chronic ischemia, vasculitis, e.g.,
    Henoch–Schonlein purpura)
  - Strictures of other origins (surgical anastomosis stricture,
    irradiation, amyloid deposition)

- Abdominal plain film can identify several signs (air–fluid
  levels, dilated loops), however it shows poor sensitivity (50–
  66 %) in the diagnosis site and origin of small bowel
  obstruction.
- CT imaging represents the imaging of choice in suspected
  small bowel obstruction. CT is reported to be very sensitive

for high-grade small bowel obstruction; however, it is less sensitive for low-grade partial obstruction.

- CT sign is represented by:
  - Small bowel dilatation (>2.5 cm)
  - Discrepant caliber at transition zone from dilated to non-dilated loop
  - "Small bowel feces sign" described as the presence of gas bubbles mixed with particulate matter (resembling the feces CT appearance) proximal to obstruction

- If the entire small bowel is dilated without the evidence of a transitional zone, the differential diagnosis with adynamic ileus should be considered.
- If the small bowel feces sign is located in the terminal ileum immediately proximal to the ileocecal valve, a bezoar should be considered as the cause of the obstruction.
- If oral iodinated contrast agent is administered, the passage of contrast material through transition zone indicates incomplete obstruction.
- Once the *site* of obstruction is identified, radiologist should pay particular attention looking for CT sign that can suggest the *cause* of obstruction.

- CT findings suggesting the cause of SBO are:
  - Soft tissue mass suggesting small bowel tumor or other sign of peritoneal carcinomatosis should be ruled out. Ileal gallstone is easily identified (usually are large calcified stone; look for pneumobilia that is commonly present due to bilioenteric fistula).
  - Bowel wall thickening can be easily detected; however, this finding itself is very nonspecific (Crohn's disease, small bowel tumor, inflammatory changes).
  - In case of adhesion, no soft tissue mass neither bowel wall thickening is visible at the level of transition zone, while the so-called fat notch sign can be distinguished.

Strangulated Small Bowel Obstruction

- In case of obstruction due to adhesion, strangulation of bowel loops may complicate the scenario (strangulated obstruction) requiring surgery urgently to reduce the risk of small bowel ischemia and following complication such as perforation and peritonitis.
- Strangulated obstruction occurs frequently in case of hernia and volvulus and in all conditions in which a "closed loop obstruction" is present (Fig. 2).

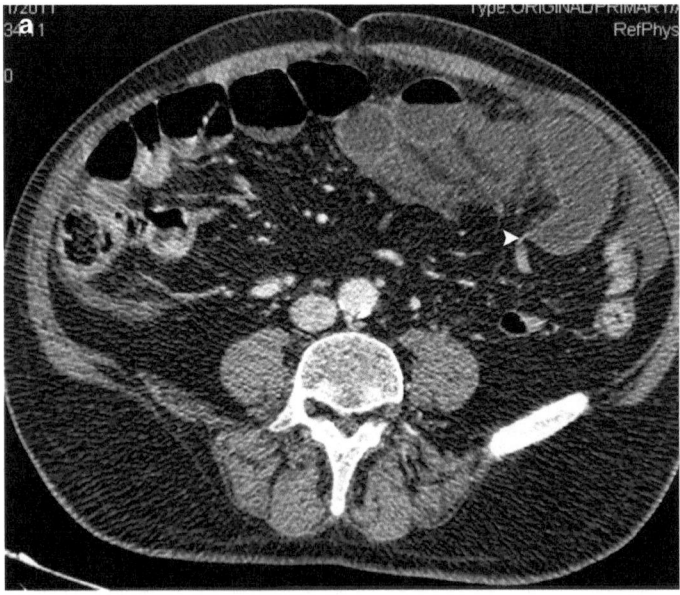

Fig. 2 (**a–c**) Show CT sign of strangulated small bowel closed loop obstruction. A group of dilated small bowel loops is visible with two different transition zones (*arrowhead* in **a** and **b**). Mesenteric fat corresponding to dilated bowel loops shows diffuse fat stranding. (**c**) A coronal MPR shows the twisted bowel loops and involvement. (**a** and **b**) Image sign of acute mesenteric critical ischemia is also visible: bowel wall of dilated loops shows poor contrast enhancement; however, no sign of pneumatosis is present

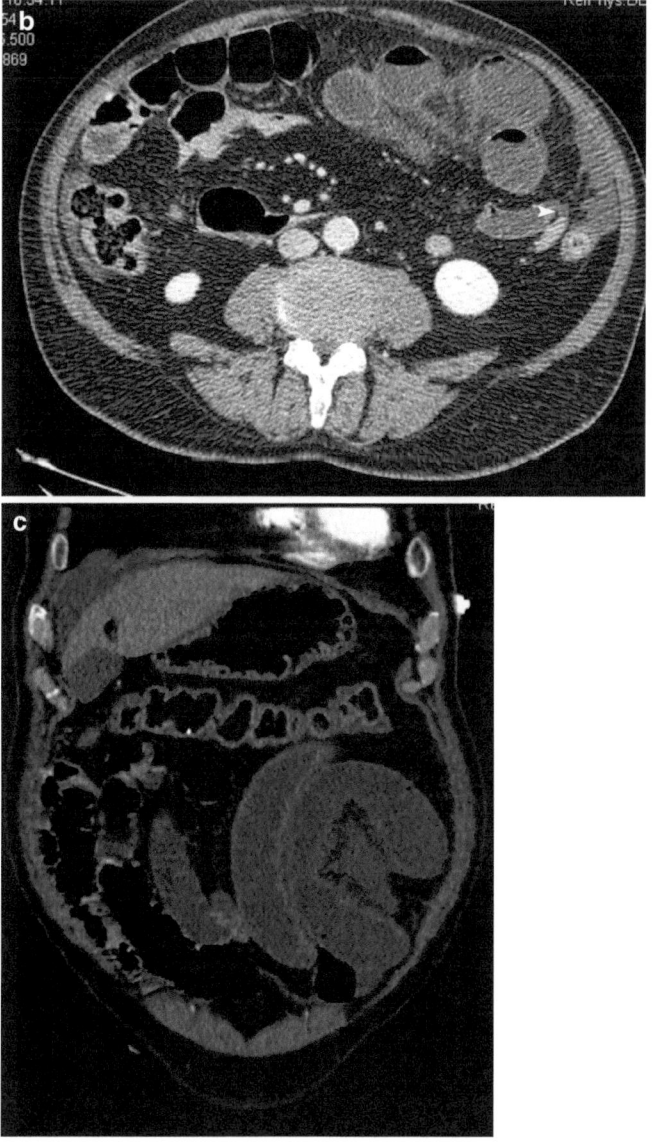

Fig. 2 (continued)

- *Closed loop obstruction* is defined as obstruction at two points along the course of the bowel at a single site with involvement of mesentery with *whirl sign* (twisting of bowel and mesentery on CT with stretched vessels converging toward the site of the obstruction).
- In case of strangulated obstruction, venous congestion of the involved loop is frequently present leading to modification of bowel wall appearance at CT.
- *Slight circumferential thickening* of bowel wall represents CT sign of strangulation with increased attenuation at unenhanced CT with stratification (*target/halo sign*).
- *Beak sign* defined as serrated beak-like narrowing at the transitional zone plus bowel wall thickening at the obstructed segment is a specific sign of closed loop obstruction with regional vascular engorgement.
- CT sign of compromise of the affected bowel wall is represented by poor or no enhancement of the bowel wall; delayed enhancement of the bowel wall due to venous engorgement; and mesenteric haziness due to edema, ascites, pneumatosis intestinalis, and gas in the portal vein (see also acute mesenteric ischemia).

Colonic Obstruction

- Colonic obstruction is caused by malignant colonic stricture, benign inflammatory stricture (diverticulitis, Crohn's disease, infective colitis), fecal impaction, or extrinsic compression (large pelvic tumor, endometriosis, pelvic abscess). Other causes of colonic obstruction are represented by colonic volvulus (sigmoid, cecum, or transverse colon is involved), colonic hernia (sigmoid colon in left inguinal hernia, diaphragmatic hernia), or adhesion.
- In colonic obstruction the small bowel may be dilated as well (incompetent ileocecal valve) or not dilated (competent ileocecal valve).

- In case of colonic obstruction, colonic dilatation is more relevant at the level of the cecum (10 cm diameter of the cecum is considered critical for impeding perforation).
- CT can easily identify the site and cause of colonic obstruction.

Suggested Reading

Silva AC, Pimenta M, Guimaraes LS (2009) Small bowel obstruction: what to look for. Radiographics 29(2):423–439

Graça BM, Freire PA, Brito JB, Ilharco JM, Carvalheiro VM, Caseiro-Alves F (2010) Gastroenterologic and radiologic approach to obscure gastrointestinal bleeding: how, why, and when? Radiographics 30(1):235–252

Delabrousse E, Sarliève P, Sailley N, Aubry S, Kastler BA (2007) Cecal volvulus: CT findings and correlation with pathophysiology. Emerg Radiol 14(6):411–415

Ha HK, Lee SH, Rha SE, Kim JH, Byun JY, Lim HK, Chung JW, Kim JG, Kim PN, Lee MG, Auh YH (2000) Radiologic features of vasculitis involving the gastrointestinal tract. Radiographics 20:779–794

Elsayes KM, Al-Hawary MM, Jagdish J, Ganesh HS, Platt JF (2010) CT enterography: principles, trends, and interpretation of findings. Radiographics 30(7):1955–1970

Goldstein N, Dulai M (2006) Contemporary morphologic definition of backwash ileitis in ulcerative colitis and features that distinguish it from Crohn disease. Am J Clin Pathol 126:365–376

Miller PA, Mezwa DG, Feczko PJ, Jafri ZH, Madrazo BL (1995) Imaging of abdominal hernias. Radiographics 15(2):333–347

Rha SE, Ha HK, Lee S-H, Kim J-H, Kim J-K, Kim JH, Kim PN, Lee M-G, Auh Y-H (2000) CT and MR imaging findings of bowel ischemia from various primary causes. Radiographics 20(1):29–42

C

Carcinoid

- The term of carcinoid tumor, first introduced by a pathologist in 1907 to designate tumor thought to be benign that looks like a carcinoma, refers in fact to very different entities. It should no longer be used. The WHO recommendations are to use the term of neuroendocrine tumor (NET) in association with the seat and degree of differentiation of the tumor. Carcinoid tumor usually refers to a well-differentiated NET of the appendix or the small bowel embryologically arising from the midgut most often localized in the ileum. Other locations of NET are the pancreas, the lung, the stomach, and, more rarely, the rectum, the esophagus, and the hypopharynx.
- Carcinoid tumors account for 25 % of all small bowel tumors, and multiple primary sites occur in 15–35 % of patients. Carcinoid tumors arise in the submucosa and grow very slowly, but all have malignant potential. Malignancy is determined by the presence of local invasion or metastatic spread, rather than histologically. Tumors smaller than 1 cm are rarely invasive, whereas those larger than 2 cm have usually metastasized by the time of diagnosis.

P. Paolantonio, C. Dromain, *Imaging of Small Bowel, Colon and Rectum*,   33
A-Z Notes in Radiological Practice and Reporting,
DOI 10.1007/978-88-470-5489-9_3, © Springer-Verlag Italia 2014

- Most of tumors are asymptomatic. However a carcinoid syndrome with flush and diarrhea occurs in 10 % of patients due to relapse of a vasoactive substance, the serotonin. The presence of a carcinoid tumor is a sign of very large tumor, with serotonin secretion that exceeds the capacity of liver metabolism, or more frequently the presence of liver metastases. In more advanced tumor, a mesenteric involvement with an important fibrotic reaction (due to serotonin secretion) may cause König syndrome and small bowel occlusion (Fig. 1). Finally, liver metastases are present in 20 % of patients at the time of diagnosis.

- CT enteroclysis is the imaging method of choice for the detection of the primary tumor allowing a good visualization of the small bowel wall as well as the extraluminal environment. Acquisition techniques must be standardized and optimized, including acquisitions at the late arterial (30 s after the beginning of injection) and portal venous (70–90 s after the beginning of injection) phases. The contribution of arterial acquisition increases sensitivity (20 % up) of the detection of liver metastases.

- CT imaging also plays a major role for the staging of the disease in association with somatostatin receptor imaging. ^{18}F-DOPA PET is the scintigraphy of choice, enabling to detect midgut NETs that produce serotonin, with a higher sensitivity than somatostatin receptor scintigraphy.

- The liver is the most common site of NET metastases. Accurate liver assessment being crucial for the prognostic and the treatment planning, a liver MRI with diffusion-weighted images is recommended to be performed in the initial morphologic assessment. Liver metastases from NET are typically hypervascularized in the arterial phase with washout.

Carcinomatosis, Peritoneal

- Peritoneal carcinomatosis (PC) is the seeding and implantation of neoplastic cells into the peritoneal cavity and represents the advanced stage of some abdominal and pelvic

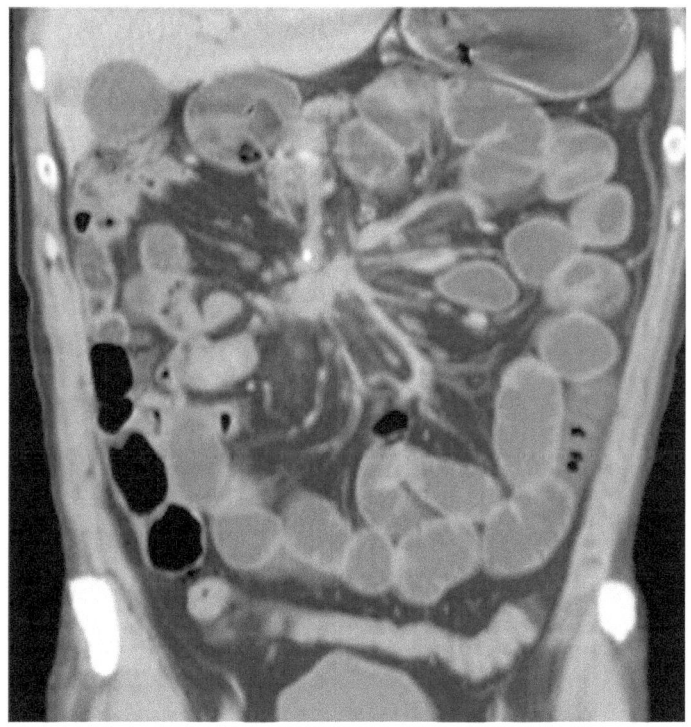

Fig. 1 Mesenteric carcinomatosis from a carcinoid tumor. Coronal reconstruction CT image shows a fibrous mesenteric mass with distorted bowel loops and dilatation of mesenteric vessels very suggestive of a mesenteric carcinomatosis from a neuroendocrine ileal tumor

tumors. Ovarian, stomach, and colorectal cancers are the most common primary tumors leading to PC.

• Recent aggressive surgical treatment with complete resection of the peritoneal implants associated with intraperitoneal chemotherapy and hyperthermy (ICHP) yields a highly significant increase of overall survival rate of 53 % at 3 years and 48.5 % at 5 years. This new aggressive surgical approach requires accurate intraperitoneal assessment of the presence or the absence of peritoneal carcinomatosis but also of the exact extent of carcinomatosis.

- CT is the imaging modality of choice for the detection of PC with an overall sensitivity ranging from 60 to 82 %. This sensitivity is depending on radiologists, tumor size, and the location of tumor deposits with lower sensitivity in lean patient without ascites, in case of infracentimetric tumor deposit and location in the pelvis, in the mesentery, or in contact with bowel loops. Different patterns of peritoneal carcinomatosis on CT imaging include ascites; tiny 1–5 mm nodules (Fig. 2a) most often localized in the greater omentum, lesser omentum, and mesentery; presence of >5 mm nodules with oval shape or a star-shaped appearance; a tissue mass which can reach sizes of several centimeters typically found in the pelvis; and irregular soft tissue thickenings of the abdominal viscera and peritoneal walls. In cases of involvement of the visceral peritoneum over small bowel loops and colonic surface, bowel distortion, bowel wall thickening, and bowel obstruction can be present. The infiltration of the greater omentum can range from increased density of fat anterior to the colon or small bowel to large masses, called omental cakes, separating the colon and small bowel from the anterior abdominal wall (Fig. 2b). Additional sign that may be related to the presence of peritoneal carcinomatosis is the appearance of a ureteral dilatation, ovary metastases, and the presence of cardiophrenic lymph nodes.

- FDG PET-CT has been reported to be useful for the detection of PC. Indeed, unlike CT, FDG PET has an excellent contrast resolution between the tumoral implant and the background signal allowing a good visibility of PC nodules. The sensitivity of PET scan varies from 63 to 93 % depending to the PC location. However FDG PET has some limitations that are small size nodules, implants with a mucinous histology, and location in the right hypochondrium. Moreover some physiologic tracer uptake into the stomach and the bowel can mimic PC and lead to false positive.

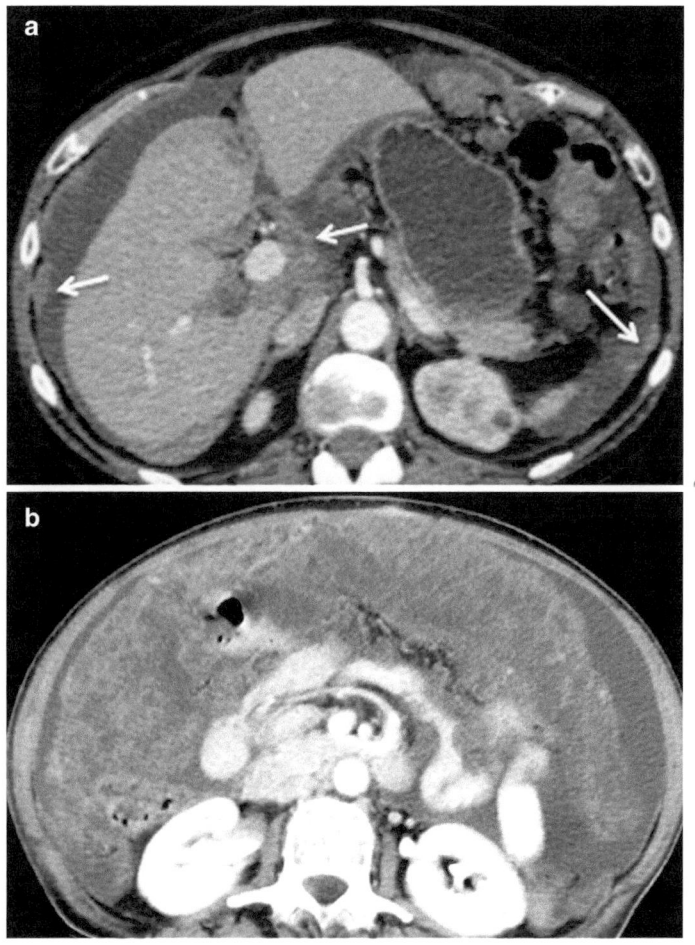

Fig. 2 (**a**) Peritoneal carcinomatosis: CT image shows ascites and tiny peritoneal nodules at the level of the peritoneal abdominal wall and lesser omentum (*arrows*). (**b**) Omental cake. Axial contrast-enhanced CT image shows a diffuse soft tissue density infiltration and thickening of the great omental fat corresponding to an advanced peritoneal carcinomatosis

- Diffusion-weighted MRI has been also reported to have a high per-lesion sensitivity for the detection of PC. Using high b value, it allows a good suppression of the signal of fat, ascites, and digestive fluid. Its per-site sensitivity ranges from 74 to 90 %. Limits are the physiologic restriction of certain organs (lymph nodes, spleen, adrenal glands) and the T2 shine-through effect as well as low-cell-density tumor and calcified tumors.

Cathartic Colon

- Cathartic colon is a functional complication due to prolonged use of stimulant or irritant laxatives resulting in neuromuscular incoordination. Some morphologic findings may suggest together with anamnestic and clinical data of the cathartic colon. Patients present with constipation, and abdominal bloating. Findings at imaging are represented by flattened and smooth colonic surface, diminished or absent haustration, "pseudostrictures" (tapered areas of narrowing due to sustained tonus of circular muscles), and shortened ascending colon. Cathartic colon usually affects elderly patients but may be also seen in younger patients as a possible complication of bulimia.

Cavitary Mesenteric Lymph Node Syndrome

- Cavitary mesenteric lymph node syndrome is a complication of celiac disease consisting in the association of enlarged lymph nodes with central cavitation within the jejunoileal mesentery, splenic atrophy, and intestinal changes of celiac disease.

CDAI

- CDAI (Crohn's Disease Activity Index) is a score of inflammatory activity used in Crohn's disease patient using clinical and laboratoristic data. CDAI is basically a research tool used to quantify the symptoms of patients with Crohn's disease. CDAI is used in research studies done on medications used to treat Crohn's disease; most major studies on newer medications use the CDAI in order to define response or remission of disease. Remission of Crohn's disease is defined as a fall in the CDAI of less than 150. Severe disease was defined as a value of greater than 450. Most major research studies on medications in Crohn's disease define response as a fall of the CDAI of greater than 70 points.

Cecal Volvulus

- Colonic volvulus is a possible cause of colonic obstruction. Volvulus of the cecum is frequently associated with colonic malrotation with a long mesentery resulting in poor fixation of the right colon. Cecum may rotate anteriorly to the ascending colon (type I or "cecal bascule") or in the left upper abdominal quadrant (type II). The volvulus is triggered usually by sudden colonic distension due to constipation and distal colonic obstruction or by trauma. Cecal volvulus may lead to vascular compromise with strangulation (see mesenteric ischemia) followed by perforation. Cecum caliber >10 cm is at risk for impending perforation or infarction.

Celiac Disease

- Celiac disease (celiac sprue or gluten-sensitive enteropathy) is a form of intestinal malabsorption due to intestinal mucosa's exposure to gluten. It is characterized by a wide spectrum of clinical presentation.
- Typical presentation of celiac disease is pediatric onset of malabsorption symptoms. However celiac disease can be diagnosed in adult patients as well. When celiac disease is suspected, lab test (anti-gliadin anti-endomysium antibodies) as well as jejunal biopsy is necessary to confirm the diagnosis. Imaging plays a second role in the diagnosis of celiac disease. Many subjects affected by celiac disease do not have any imaging findings.
- Using dedicated imaging study for the small bowel (MR/CT enterography/enteroclysis), some findings suggesting the diagnosis of celiac disease can be detected. These findings are represented by jejunal fold flattening and ileal jejunization (more than threefolds for inch) as well as the combination of both previous findings (so-called intestinal reversal fold pattern). Celiac patients can also present with increased intestinal loop's caliber (>2.5 cm) without a definite transition zone due to intestinal atony. Complicating lesions of celiac disease are represented by transient intussusceptions (due to intestinal atony), hyposplenism, and ascites. In long-standing celiac disease, an increased risk of intestinal lymphoma is described. Therefore bowel wall thickening in celiac patients is suspected for intestinal lymphoma.

Chronic Inflammatory Bowel Disease

- Chronic inflammatory bowel diseases are represented by *Crohn's disease* and *ulcerative colitis*. In children a third form, the so-called indeterminate-type colitis, is also described. Differential diagnosis between Crohn's disease and ulcerative findings requires combination of clinical findings, endoscopic and histological results, as well as imaging findings. Imaging plays a crucial role in the study of the small bowel that is frequently involved in Crohn's disease while is spared in ulcerative colitis.

- Imaging techniques for small bowel imaging are represented by conventional barium studies, dedicated US study (SICUS), and CT/MR enterography/enteroclysis.
- Indeterminate-type colitis is a form of chronic inflammatory disease in children with no definite finding of Crohn's disease nor ulcerative colitis and it is thought to be a transient form of chronic inflammation in children.

Cobblestone Appearance

- Cobblestone appearance is a characteristic radiologic and gross appearance of the intestinal mucosa in Crohn's disease, due to submucosal involvement and to severe ulcerative disease with crisscrossing of the ulcers through inflamed but intact mucosa; intestinal "cobblestoning" may also occur in ulcerative colitis – where ulcers alternate with regenerating mucosa.

Colon Carcinoma

- Colon adenocarcinoma is the most common type of gastrointestinal cancer. It begins in the cells of glandular structures in the inner layer of the colon and spreads first into the wall of the colon and potentially into the lymphatic system and other organs.

- Most colon cancer is sporadic, but hereditary mutation of the APC gene is the cause of familial adenomatous polyposis and hereditary non-polyposis colon cancer syndrome (HNPCC, Lynch syndrome). Inflammatory bowel disease such as ulcerative colitis and Crohn's disease also carry an increased risk of developing colorectal adenocarcinoma.
- The incidence of colorectal cancer peaks at about age 65 years equal for males and females.
- Colon adenocarcinoma progresses slowly and may not present symptoms for up to 5 years. It is now often detected during screening procedures. Other common clinical presentations include iron-deficiency anemia, rectal bleeding, abdominal pain, change in bowel habits, and intestinal obstruction or perforation. Right-sided lesions are more likely to bleed and cause diarrhea, while left-sided tumors are usually detected later and could present with bowel obstruction.
- The initial diagnosis is usually made with colonoscopy with biopsy confirmation of cancer tissue.
- CT imaging is not routinely performed for the detection of cancer colon but is more used for the preoperative staging to rule out lymph nodes and metastases. Colorectal cancer typically appears as a soft tissue mass that narrows the colonic lumen. It can also manifest as focal colonic wall thickening and luminal narrowing. CT imaging also assesses the local extension of the tumor (infiltration of pericolic fat, loss of fat planes, or invasion of adjacent organs) and distant metastases in the liver, lung, peritoneum, and abdominal lymph nodes. Complications such as obstruction, perforation, and fistula can be readily visualized with CT.
- Positron emission tomography (PET) scans are indicated during follow-up in case of suspected recurrence and elevation of blood marker like CEA and whenever a major surgical decision is discussed.

Crohn's Disease

- Crohn's disease is a chronic inflammatory bowel disease that may affect the entire bowel with a predominant involvement of the small bowel and colon. The terminal ileum is the most commonly involved segment. The diagnosis of Crohn's disease is based on the combination of clinical findings, endoscopic and histological results, and imaging findings. Imaging plays a crucial role in the diagnosis as well as follow-up of Crohn's disease.
- Modern imaging of Crohn's disease is performed using MR/CT enterography/enteroclysis in the assessment of small bowel Crohn's disease and pelvic MRI in the assessment of perianal Crohn's disease, while for colonic localization optical colonoscopy remains the standard reference.
- CT/MRI findings of Crohn's disease are represented by small *bowel wall thickening* with a segmentary involvement of the bowel and presence of *deep ulcers* leading to *cobblestone appearance*. Inflammatory process involved the entire small bowel wall as well as perivisceral fat with the so-called fibrofatty proliferation (thickened perivisceral fat with bowel loops separation, engorgement of vasa recta with the so-called comb sign).
- Bowel wall thickening may lead to lumen narrowing and *intestinal strictures*.
- *Skip intestinal segment* between involved loops with narrowed lumen usually shows increased luminal caliber with pseudosacculation (Fig. 3).
- During active disease, thickened bowel wall shows increased *contrast enhancement* with different possible pattern (transmural or layered enhancement) (Fig. 4).

In case of fibrotic disease, the degree of contrast enhancement is reduced with respect to normal bowel wall during the enteric phase (70 s after contrast medium administration).

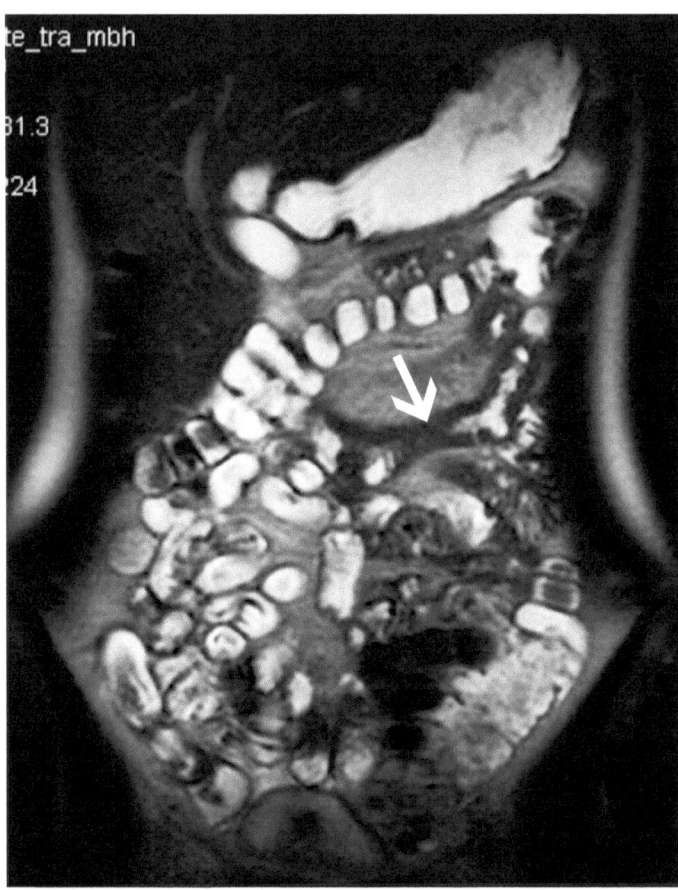

Fig. 3 Coronal T2-weighted images from an MR enterography study in a 22-year-old patient affected by Crohn's disease. *Arrow* indicates an affected jejunal segment presenting with asymmetric wall thickening, pseudosacculation, deep ulcers, and fibrofatty proliferation (see separation between affected loop and transverse colon due to adipose pseudomass)

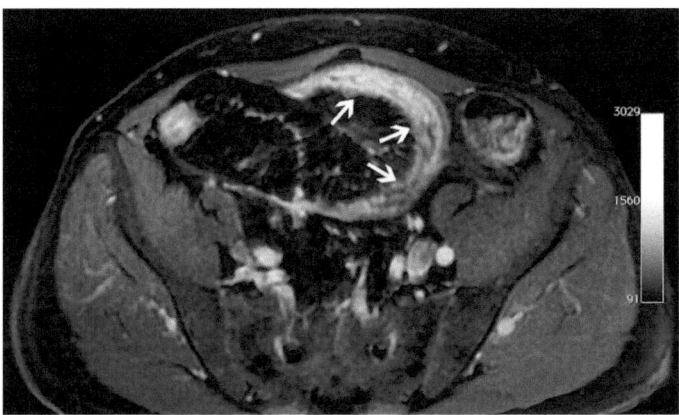

Fig. 4 Contrast-enhanced T1-weighted image from an MR enterography in a patient with active ileal Crohn's disease. *Arrows* indicate a long affected ileal segment with mural thickening, layered enhancement (high signal intensity in the inner bowel wall layer and less enhancement in the outer one). Ulcers and engorged vasa recta (*comb sign*) are visible as well

- MRI is preferred to assess Crohn's disease activity due to its ability to better distinguish between *edema* and *fibrosis* showing high and low signal intensity on T2-weighted images, respectively. Strictures, abscess, and fistulas represent complicating lesions of Crohn's disease.
- First diagnosis of Crohn's disease based on imaging findings alone is nearly impossible requiring integration of clinical endoscopic and histological findings.
- Many inflammatory processes of the small and large bowel in the acute or subacute phase and also some neoplasm may mimic Crohn's disease at imaging.

  Differential diagnosis should consider *infective diseases*, Yersinia (usually in the terminal ileum, resolves in 3–4 months), tuberculosis (more severe involvement of the cecum and associated with pulmonary TBC), actinomycosis, histoplasmosis, blastomycosis, and anisakiasis; segmental infarction (acute onset, elderly patients); radiation ileitis (appropriate history); *lymphoma* (no spasm, no strictures, or string sign; luminal narrowing is uncommon); *carcinoid tumor* (tumor nodules); eosinophilic gastroenteritis; and *intestinal vasculitis* (Henoch–Schonlein purpura).

Colonic Ulcer

- Possible causes of colonic ulcers are represented by the following: chronic inflammatory bowel disease (ulcerative colitis, Crohn's disease); ischemic (ischemic colitis); traumatic (radiation injuries, caustic colitis); neoplastic (primary colonic carcinoma, metastases); inflammatory (pseudomembranous colitis, diverticulitis, Behcet disease, solitary rectal ulcer, nonspecific benign ulceration); and infection – protozoan (amebiasis, schistosomiasis, strongyloidiasis), bacterial (salmonellosis, tuberculosis, Yersinia colitis, staphylococcal colitis, campylobacter), fungal (histoplasmosis, actinomycosis, candidiasis), and viral (herpes proctocolitis, CMV).

CT Colonography

- CT colonography or virtual colonoscopy is a novel imaging study of the colon. CT colonography requires bowel preparation using cathartic ages and/or tagging agents (oral iodinated contrast medium) and bowel distension obtained by means of colonic insufflations by means of rectal tube.
- CT acquisition is performed using thin collimation without intravenous contrast medium injection with patient in prone and supine position.
- Post-processing is crucial in imaging interpretation that presents benefit by the combination of 2D data set, MPR reconstruction, and 3D VR or SSD reconstruction with endoluminal

views. Dedicated software are suited for virtual colonoscopy post-processing and imaging review on commercially available workstation helping radiologist in reporting virtual colonoscopy by analyzing CT data set using post-processing tools. Moreover CAD applications dedicated to CT colonography are also available useful to reduce false-negative rates in nonexpert readers. Colonic strictures, tumors, and diverticular disease are easily detected at virtual colonoscopy. An excellent diagnostic accuracy is also reported for detection of clinical relevant polyps (>10 mm) (Fig. 5). Differential

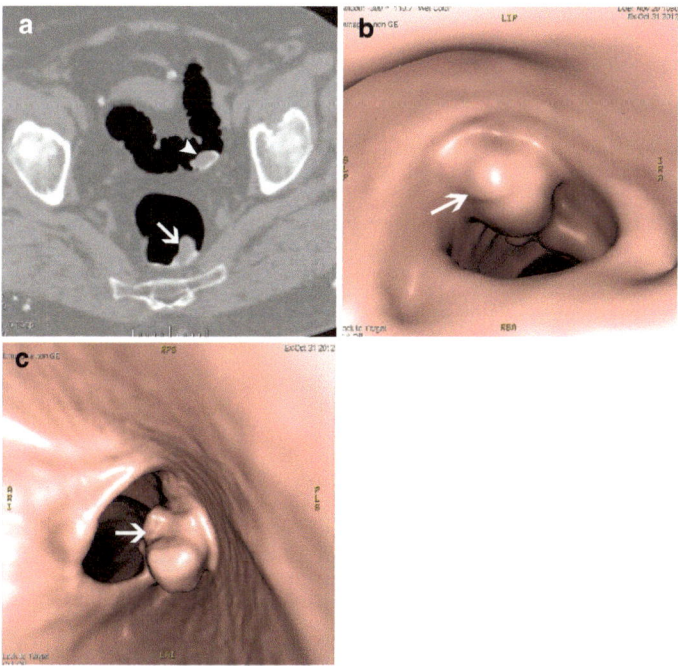

Fig. 5 Images from a CT colonography examination. (**a**) An axial CT supine scan is presented showing two significant sessile polyps at the level of the sigmoid colon (*arrowheads*) and rectum (*arrow*). (**b** and **c**) 3D VR similar endoscopic images of sigmoid and rectal polyp (*arrow*) are shown

diagnosis between colonic polyp and residual stools is based on the following criteria: stools usually change position between prone and supine scans; using fluid tagging stools are usually marked by the tagging agent; and stools are often homogeneous with tiny internal air bubbles.

- Clinical indications to virtual colonoscopy are represented by incomplete optical colonoscopy (Fig. 6), assessment of diverticular disease, and colonic examination in frail and elderly patients. Virtual colonoscopy can also be proposed as screening method in patients unwilling to undergo optical colonoscopy. Inflammatory bowel disease does not represent an indication to virtual colonoscopy examination.

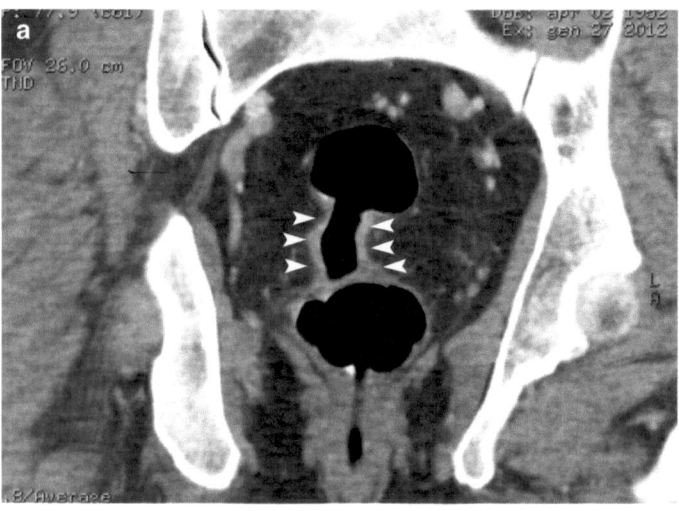

Fig. 6 A case of a patient with incomplete optical colonoscopy due to stricturing rectal carcinoma. Patient underwent virtual colonoscopy showing the rectal carcinoma (**a**) presenting with focal mural thickening (*arrowheads*) and lumen narrowing and an apple core appearance; in the same patients a synchronous colonic carcinoma was identified by virtual colonoscopy at the level of the cecum (**b**) with similar CT appearance (*arrowheads*)

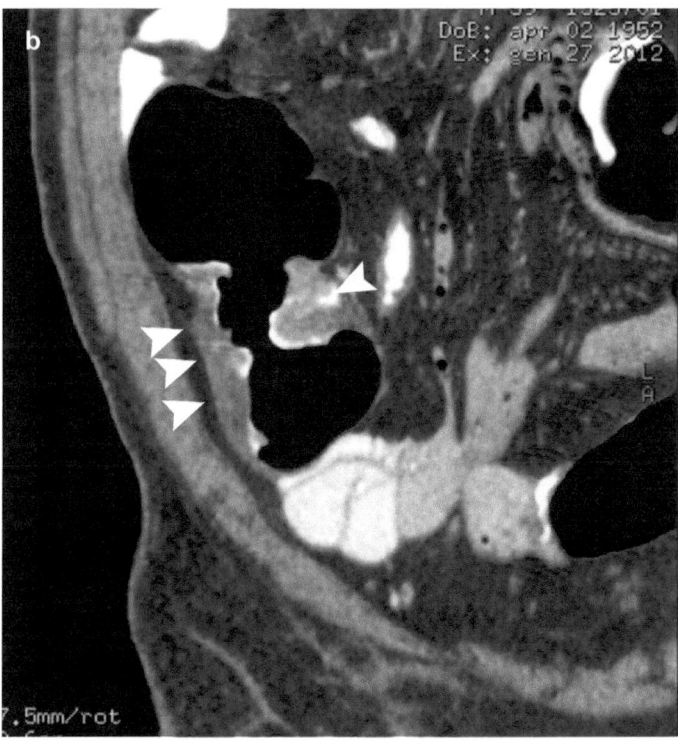

Fig. 6 (continued)

CT Enteroclysis/Enterography

- CT enterography and CT enteroclysis represent dedicated CT study of the small bowel based on CT dynamic study of a well-distended small bowel. In CT enteroclysis bowel distension is achieved by means of jejunal intubation and continuous fluid administration (usually water) at high flow rate to obtain reflex intestinal atony.

On the other hand, CT enterography is a valid alternative to CT enteroclysis; it is less invasive since bowel distension is achieved by means of oral fluid overload using hypodense non-absorbable or hyperosmolar solution (PEG or mannitol solution). In adult 1.5 l of PEG solution administered 20 min before imaging acquisition is suggested to achieve adequate bowel distension. CT protocol is based on a multiphasic study using thin collimation and MPR reconstruction on coronal plane.

• Unenhanced study is mandatory in patients with suspected GI bleeding. Dynamic study is suggested to assess in a single exam mesenteric vessels as well as bowel wall. Contrast-enhanced CT protocol should include arterial phase and enteric phase (70 s after contrast medium injection) to study small bowel wall enhancement. Dose reduction systems (tube current modulation) are suggested especially in Crohn's disease patients that underwent several CT studies along their life.

CT Perfusion

• CT perfusion is a CT acquisition technique based on stable table CT acquisition during contrast medium administration and on dedicated post-processing leading to quantitative assessment of perfusion parameters (blood volume, blood flow, mean transit time, and mean permeability surface). These parameters can be used in research settings to assess tumor perfusion.

Suggested Reading

Best WR, Becktel JM, Singleton JW, Kern F Jr (1976) Development of a Crohn's disease activity index. National Cooperative Crohn's Disease Study. Gastroenterology 70(3):439–444

Dahnert W (2002) Radiology review manual, 5th edn. Lippincott and Williams, Philadelphia

Delabrousse E, Sarliève P, Sailley N, Aubry S, Kastler BA (2007 Nov) Cecal volvulus: CT findings and correlation with pathophysiology. Emerg Radiol 14(6):411–415

Dighe S, Castellano E, Blake H, Jeyadevan N, Koh MU, Orten M, Swift I, Brown G (2012) Perfusion CT to assess angiogenesis in colon cancer: technical limitations and practical challenges. Br J Radiol 85(1018): e814–e825

Dromain C, Leboulleux S, Auperin A, Goere D, Malka D, Lumbroso J, Schumberger M, Sigal R, Elias D (2008) Staging of peritoneal carcinomatosis: enhanced CT vs. PET/CT. Abdom Imaging 33:87–93

Kawaguchi T, Takazoe M (2012 Feb) Natural history and prognosis of inflammatory bowel diseases. Nihon Rinsho 70(Suppl 1):48–51

Laghi A, Paolantonio P, Iafrate F, Borrelli O, Dito L, Tomei E, Cucchiara S, Passariello R (2003) MR of the small bowel with a biphasic oral contrast agent (polyethylene glycol): technical aspects and findings in patients affected by Crohn's disease. Radiol Med 106(1–2):18–27

Laghi A, Paolantonio P, Passariello R (2005) Small bowel. Magn Reson Imaging Clin N Am 13(2):331–348, Review

Lin CY, Chua SK, Wanf SH, Tai WC, Wang CC (2013) Primary small bowel malignancy: a 10-year clinical experience from Southern Taiwan. Hepatogastroenterology 60(124):756–758

Macari M, Bini EJ, Jacobs SL, Lange N, Lui YW (2003) Filling defects at CT colonography: pseudo- and diminutive lesions (the good), polyps (the bad), flat lesions, masses, and carcinomas (the ugly). Radiographics 23(5):1073–1091

Paolantonio P, Tomei E, Rengo M, Ferrari R, Lucchesi P, Laghi A (2007) Adult celiac disease: MRI findings. Abdom Imaging 32(4):433–440, Review

Paulsen SR, Huprich JE, Fletcher JG, Booya F, Young BM, Fidler JL, Daniel Johnson C, Barlow JM, Earnest F IV (2006) CT enterography as a diagnostic tool in evaluating small bowel disorders: review of clinical experience with over 700 cases. Radiographics 26(3):641–657

Paulson EK, McDermott VG, Keogan MT, DeLong DM, Frederick MG, Nelson RC (1998) Carcinoid metastases to the liver: role of triple-phase helical CT. Radiology 206:143–150

Pickhardt PJ (2004) Differential diagnosis of polypoid lesions seen at CT colonography (virtual colonoscopy). Radiographics 24(6):1535–1556

Regge D, Della Monica P, Galatola G, Laudi C, Zambon A, Correale L, Asnaghi R, Barbaro B, Borghi C, Campanella D, Cassinis MC, Ferrari R, Ferraris A, Hassan C, Iafrate F, Iussich G, Laghi A, Massara R, Neri

E, Sali L, Venturini S, Gandini G (2013 Jan) Efficacy of computer-aided detection as a second reader for 6–9-mm lesions at CT colonography: multicenter prospective trial. Radiology 266(1):168–176

Rha SE, Ha HK, Lee S-H, Kim J-H, Kim J-K, Kim JH, Kim PN, Lee M-G, Auh Y-H (2000) CT and MR imaging findings of bowel ischemia from various primary causes. Radiographics 20(1):29–42

Rubesin SE, Saul SH, Laufer I, Levine MS (1985) Carpet lesions of the colon. Radiographics 5(4):537–552

Soussan M, Des Guetz G, Barrau V, Aflalo-Hazan V, Pop G, Mehanna Z, Rust E, Aparicio T, Douard R, Benamouzig R, Wind P, Eder V (2012 Jul) Comparison of FDG-PET/CT and MR with diffusion-weighted imaging for assessing peritoneal carcinomatosis from gastrointestinal malignancy. Eur Radiol 22(7):1479–1487

D

Defecography, MR

- MR defecography is a study of the pelvis composed by a morphologic study and by a dynamic study dedicated to the functional pelvic floor disease.
- MR protocol requires patient preparation (rectal cleansing by means of enema) and rectal distension by means of sonographic gel injected through a rectal tube.

  Phase array is used for signal reception. Patient is positioned in supine position.
- Morphologic study consists in high-resolution T2-weighted sequences acquired on axial, coronal, and sagittal planes in order to study morphologic features of pelvic floor and sphincter complex.
- Dynamic study is based on the acquisition of dynamic high-contrast high temporal resolution sequences, fast imaging with steady-state precession (FISP, balanced FFE, FIESTA) sequence. Single-slice sagittal FISP sequence with high temporal resolution is acquired continuously over 40 s time period at rest and during patient straining and defecation.

P. Paolantonio, C. Dromain, *Imaging of Small Bowel, Colon and Rectum*, 53
A-Z Notes in Radiological Practice and Reporting,
DOI 10.1007/978-88-470-5489-9_4, © Springer-Verlag Italia 2014

Descending Perineum Syndrome

- Descending perineum syndrome refers to a condition where the perineum descends below the bony outlet of the pelvis during straining and defecation due to weakness of the pelvic floor muscle and excessive straining during defecation. Descending perineum syndrome can be complicated by protrusion of pelvic organs (rectal prolapse and rectocele, colpocele, enterocele, and cystocele) leading to several symptoms including chronic constipation due to "obstructed defecation" (secondary to rectal prolapse and rectocele).
- Descending perineum syndrome can be studied using MR defecography. An MR defecography is useful to describe the position of pelvic organs with respect to an imaginary line drawn from the inferior aspect of the pubic symphysis to the last coccygeal vertebra, the so-called pubococcygeal line.

Diverticulosis of the Colon

- Colonic diverticulosis is a common condition represented by the presence of multiple colonic pseudodiverticula (acquired herniation of mucosa and submucosa through the muscularis propria). Frequently colonic diverticulosis is associated with constipation and hypertrophy of muscular colonic layer and haustral hypertrophy.
- Diverticulosis can be *asymptomatic* or leading to symptoms due to microperforation of diverticula followed by inflammatory changes of pericolic fat and colonic wall with possible abscess formation (*acute diverticulitis* and *complicated acute diverticulitis*). Several episodes of diverticulitis may hesitate into colonic wall fibrosis, stiffness, and lumen reduction with *colonic benign strictures.*
- In western countries the most common colonic segment involved in diverticular disease is represented by the sigmoid

colon, while in eastern countries right-side diverticulitis is a common condition.

- CT represent the imaging of choice in case of suspected acute diverticulitis owing to its ability to easily detect extraluminal air and inflammatory changes into the colonic wall and pericolic fat with the so-called pericolic fat stranding. In non-acute diverticular disease, CT colonography can be used to assess location and extension of diverticular disease and colonic strictures and to evaluate accurately colonic segments proximal to a diverticular colonic stricture.

DWI

- Diffusion-weighted imaging (DWI) is a functional MR imaging sequence used to identify and assess quantitatively the random motion of water molecules in human tissue. Since the cellular membrane represents a barrier to the random motion of water molecule, DWI can be used as surrogate marker of tissue cellularity. Using post-processing analysis of native DWI, data set quantitative assessment of water diffusion movement can be calculated by measuring the so-called apparent diffusion coefficient (ADC). Thanks to its ability to assess tissue cellularity, DWI was recently proposed to tumor imaging, and in gastrointestinal imaging, DWI seems to be a promising tool in rectal cancer imaging.

Suggested Reading

Chandarana H, Taouli B (2010) Diffusion-weighted MRI and liver metastases. Magn Reson Imaging Clin N Am 18(3):451–464

Seynaeve P, Billiet I, Vossaert P, Verleyen P, Steegmans A (2006) MR imaging of the pelvic floor. JBR 89:182–189

Urban BA, Fishman EK (2000) Tailored helical CT evaluation of acute abdomen. Radiographics 20(3):725–749

E

Endometriosis, GI

- Endometriosis is a gynecologic disease consisting in ectopic foci of the endometrium with recurrent bleeding, and it is responsible of chronic pelvic pain in female. Ectopic endometrium frequently is located in the annex or along uterine ligaments and in the Douglas pouch. Other locations of pelvic endometriosis are represented by the rectovaginal septum, rectal wall, and sigmoid and small bowel serosa. In such cases endometriosis can present with small implants on the serosa or can evolve in chronic inflammatory disease followed by pelvic adhesion and fibrosis. In a more invalidating pattern called deep pelvic endometriosis, large fibrotic nodules or ill-defined fibrotic masses present an infiltrative pattern from the serosa to the muscular layer to the submucosa of the gut with possible luminal narrowing.
- Pelvic MRI is the technique of choice in the assessment of pelvic endometriosis involving the gut, thanks to its ability to differentiate soft tissue. Usually deep pelvic endometriosis involving the gut presents at MRI a diffuse or focal infiltrative tissue with low signal intensity on T2-weighted images due to

P. Paolantonio, C. Dromain, *Imaging of Small Bowel, Colon and Rectum*, 57
A-Z Notes in Radiological Practice and Reporting,
DOI 10.1007/978-88-470-5489-9_5, © Springer-Verlag Italia 2014

the predominant fibrotic components. However T1-weighted images with fat saturation are also useful to distinguish small high-signal foci within fibrotic tissue due to accumulation of hemoglobin degradation products. Laparoscopy represents the gold standard for pelvic endometriosis diagnosis allowing also treatments of adhesions and ablation of small peritoneal implants.

Enteric Cyst

• Enteric cyst is a congenital cyst lined by gastrointestinal mucosa without bowel wall due to migration of small bowel or colonic diverticulum into the mesentery or mesocolon. Enteric cyst appears at cross-sectional imaging as a unilocular cystic mass with well-defined thin wall into the mesentery or mesocolon.

Enteritis

• Enteritis is an inflammation of the small bowel commonly due to ingestion of food contaminated by pathogenic micro-organism leading to abdominal pain, cramping, diarrhea, dehydration, and fever. Other forms of enteritis are represented by Crohn's disease, enteric manifestation of vasculitis, and radiation-induced enteritis.

Enteroclysis (CT/MRI)

• CT enteroclysis and MRI enteroclysis are dedicated studies of the small bowel based on small bowel distension achieved by large-volume fluid administration through a nasojejunal tube (see CT enteroclysis and MR enteroclysis).

Enterography (CT/MRI)

- CT enterography and MR enterography are dedicated studies of the small bowel based on small bowel distension achieved by oral administration of intestinal contrast medium (see CT/MR enterography).

Eosinophilic Gastroenteritis

- Eosinophilic gastroenteritis is an uncommon self-limited form of gastroenteritis with remissions plus exacerbations characterized by infiltration of eosinophilic leukocytes into the stomach and/or small bowel wall with marked peripheral eosinophilia. At cross-sectional imaging, the affected bowel presents diffuse wall thickening with possible enlarged gastric and jejunal folds, luminal narrowing, and wall rigidity. If the serosa is involved, patients present with ascites. Common sites are represented by the antrum and jejunum. Differential diagnosis should be performed with lymphoma and carcinoma.

Extrasphincteric Fistula

- Extrasphincteric fistula is a form of perianal fistula. Following Parks classification, perianal fistulas are categorized as intersphincteric, transsphincteric, suprasphincteric, and extrasphincteric. The classification is based on the relationships between the fistulous tract and the external sphincter muscle (see fistula in ano).

Suggested Reading

Amzallag-Bellenger E, Oudjit A, Ruiz A, Cadiot G, Soyer PA, Hoeffel CC
    (2012) Effectiveness of MR enterography for the assessment of small-
    bowel diseases beyond Crohn disease. Radiographics 32(5):1423–1444
Dahnert W (2002) Radiology review manual, 5th edn. Lippincott Williams,
    Philadelphia
Elsayes KM, Al-Hawary MM, Jagdish J, Ganesh HS, Platt JF (2010) CT
    enterography: principles, trends, and interpretation of findings.
    Radiographics 30(7):1955–1970
Gidwaney R, Badler RL, Yam BL, Hines JJ, Alexeeva V, Donovan V, Katz
    DS (2012) Endometriosis of abdominal and pelvic wall scars: multimo-
    dality imaging findings, pathologic correlation, and radiologic mimics.
    Radiographics 32(7):2031–2043
Maàmouri N, Guellouz S, Belkahla N, Mohsni B, Naija N, Chouaib S,
    Chaabouni H, Ben MN (2012) Eosinophilic gastroenteritis. Rev Med
    Interne 33(8):421–425
Macari M, Balthazar EJ (2001) CT of bowel wall thickening: significance
    and pitfalls of interpretation. AJR Am J Roentgenol 176:1105–1116
Maglinte D (2013) Fluoroscopic and CT enteroclysis: evidence-based clini-
    cal update. Radiol Clin North Am 51(1):149–176
Maglinte DDT, Sandrasegaran K, Lappas JC, Chiorean M (2007) CT
    enteroclysis. Radiology 245(3):661–671
O'Malley RB, Al-Hawary MM, Kaza RK, Wasnik AP, Liu PS, Hussain HK
    (2012) Rectal imaging: part 2, Perianal fistula evaluation on pelvic MRI:
    what the radiologist needs to know. AJR Am J Roentgenol 199(1):
    W43–W53
Prassopoulos P, Papanikolaou N, Grammatikakis J, Rousomoustakaki M,
    Maris T, Gourtsoyiannis N (2001) MR enteroclysis imaging of Crohn
    disease. Radiographics 21(suppl 1):S161–S172

F

Fat Stranding

- Fat stranding represents important CT findings leading radiologist attention to the site of abdominal pathology especially in patients presenting with acute abdominal pain. Fat stranding refers to an *abnormal increased attenuation in fat* (in the mesentery, omentum, retroperitoneum, or subcutaneous fat).
- The underlying pathophysiologic process is increased *edema and engorgement of lymphatics*. Abdominal fat stranding can produce various appearances:

  - *Ground-glass pattern* due to mild inflammation (subtle hazy increased attenuation of the fat).
  - *Reticulonodular pattern* due to more severe inflammation (linear areas of increased attenuation.) A reticulonodular appearance can also be observed frequently in association with neoplastic disease (fat infiltration or peritoneal carcinomatosis).

P. Paolantonio, C. Dromain, *Imaging of Small Bowel, Colon and Rectum*,   61
A-Z Notes in Radiological Practice and Reporting,
DOI 10.1007/978-88-470-5489-9_6, © Springer-Verlag Italia 2014

• *Fat stranding* is not a specific sign of a certain disease since it may occur in several conditions (appendicitis, cholecystitis, colitis, Crohn's disease, diverticulitis, epiploic appendagitis, enteritis, infiltrative carcinoma, intestinal vasculitis, mesenteric ischemia, omental infarction, omental cake, panniculitis, pancreatitis, pelvic inflammatory disease, peritoneal carcinomatosis, urologic disease, and other less common conditions). Therefore it is essential to search other findings in the region where fat stranding is present in order to reach the correct diagnosis.

Fat Notch Sign

• Fat notch sign is a recently described CT finding occulting in case of small bowel obstruction due to adhesive band. Fat notch sign corresponds to the extrinsic compression of the bowel at the transition zone by an extraluminal adhesive band (Fig. 1).

Fecal Calprotectin Protein

• Fecal calprotectin protein is a biochemical surrogate marker of chronic inflammatory bowel disease. It is a calcium- and zinc-binding protein with bacteriostatic properties abundant in neutrophil's cytosol. It is resistant to enzymatic degradation and can be easily measured in feces. In inflammatory bowel disease patients, neutrophils influx into the bowel lumen leading to increases of fecal calprotectin. On the other hand, fecal calprotectin does not increase in patients with irritable bowel syndrome.

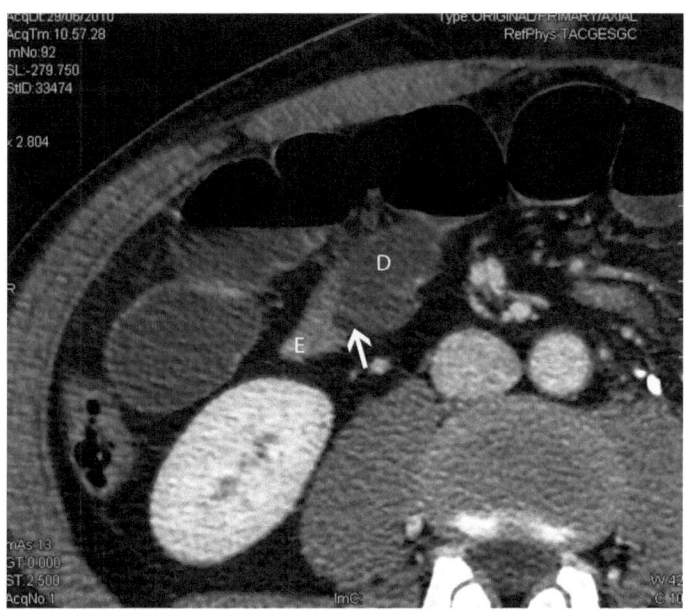

Fig. 1 The image shows a detail of a CT scan in a patient with mechanical small bowel obstruction due to adhesive band. *D* dilated small bowel loop, *E* empty small bowel loop, the *arrow* indicates the transition zone with the evidence of fat notch sign

Feces Sign (Small Bowel)

- Small bowel feces sign is a CT finding in patients with small bowel occlusion. It is defined by the presence of particulate (colon-like) feculent matter mingled with gas bubbles in the lumen of dilated loops of the small intestine. The particulate feculent material mingled with gas bubbles seen in the small bowel feces sign resembles the appearance of stool in the colon on CT scans. It is the result of delayed intestinal transit and is believed to be caused by incompletely digested food, bacterial overgrowth, or increased water absorption of the distal small bowel contents due to obstruction.

Femoral Hernia

Femoral hernia is a subtype of external hernia with bowel extending outside the abdominal cavity through the femoral canal, medial to the femoral vein. Femoral hernia is less common with respect to the inguinal hernia, is more frequent in females, and presents higher risk of complication (incarceration) due to small hernia orifice.

Fistula In Ano

- Fistula in ano origins usually from a cryptic abscess of rectal glands present in the intersphincteric space. Abscess may have spontaneous drainage with perianal fistulas.
- Based on relationship between the fistulous tract and anal sphincter complex structures, perianal fistulas were categorized by Parks into intersphincteric, transsphincteric, extrasphincteric, or suprasphincteric (Fig. 2).
- MRI of perianal region is an accurate tool in the study of perianal abscess and fistulas owing to its ability to obtain excellent anatomical details of perianal sphincter complex on TSE T2-weighted images and optimal contrast resolution for fluid collection on fat-suppressed T2-weighted images. In case of complex fistulous disease or in distinguishing active fistulous tract from inactive fibrotic fistulas after medical therapy, additional information may be given by contrast-enhanced T1-weighted fat-suppressed images. Acquisition planes should be oriented with respect to the main axes of the

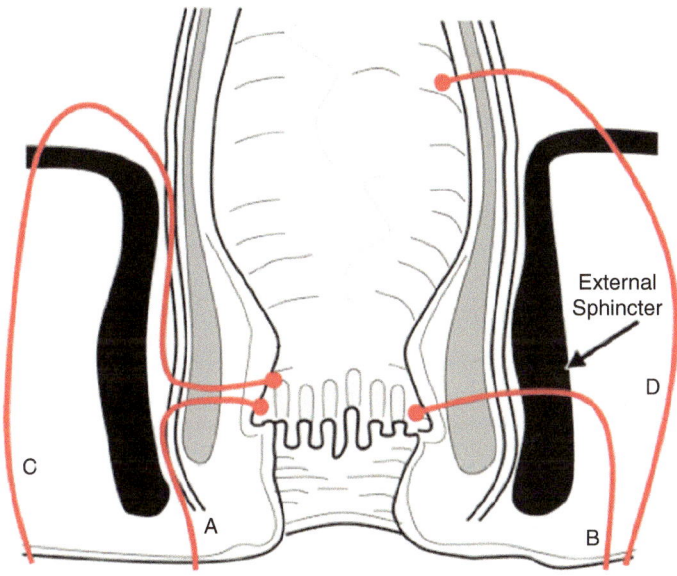

Fig. 2 Graphic illustrates the Parks classification of fistula in ano. *A* intersphincteric fistula, *B* transsphincteric fistula, *C* suprasphincteric fistula, *D* extrasphincteric fistula

anal canal (oblique axial plane, oblique coronal plane, and true sagittal plane).

FOBT

- Fecal occult blood test (FOBT) is used as screening method for colorectal cancer prevention. Different tests have been proposed to check hidden blood in the stool. The fecal immunochemical testing using specific antibodies to detect globin is preferred than the conventional guaiac test. However with both tests positive stools may result from the upper or lower gastrointestinal tract (from the mouth to the colon).

- Considering the impact of FOBT in selecting patients for further examination such as optical colonoscopy or virtual colonoscopy, it is accepted that patients with familiarity for colon cancer and positive FOBT show a high chance to have significant colonic polyp or cancer; therefore in such patients optical colonoscopy might be preferred with respect to virtual colonoscopy.

Suggested Reading

Bunn SK, Bisset WM, Main MJC, Golden BE (2001) Frecal calprotectin as a measure of disease activity in childhood inflammatory Bowel disease. J Pediatr Gastroenterol Nutr 32(2):171–177

Delabrousse E, Lubrano J, Jehl J, Morati P, Rouget C, Mantion GA, Kastler BA (2009) Small-bowel obstruction from adhesive bands and matted adhesions: CT differentiation. AJR 192:693–697

Fuchsjager MH (2002) The small-bowel feces sign. Radiology 225: 378–379

Morris J, Spencer JA, Simon N (2000) Ambrose for patient management. Radiographics 20(3):623–635

O'Malley RB, Al-Hawary MM, Kaza RK, Wasnik AP, Liu PS, Hussain HK (2012) Rectal imaging: part 2, Perianal fistula evaluation on pelvic MRI–what the radiologist needs to know. AJR Am J Roentgenol 199(1):W43–W53

Thornton E, Mendiratta-Lala M, Siewert B, Eisenberg RL (2011) Patterns of fat stranding. AJR Am J Roentgenol 197(1):W1–W14

G

Gallstone Ileus

- Gallstone ileus represents up to 5 % of small bowel obstruction more frequent in women over 60 years old with previous gallbladder disease.
- Small bowel obstruction in gallstone ileus is due to the impaction of a big gallbladder stone along the small bowel loops after a migration of gallstone from the gallbladder to the intestine through a bilioenteric fistula.
- CT sign can depict indirect sign of bilioenteric fistulas such as gas in biliary tree and collapsed gallbladder and can directly depict the presence of a calcified gallstone at the transition zone (Fig. 1).

Gas in Portal Vein

- Gas in portal vein should be considered a life-threatening event and sign of bowel infarction and gangrene until proved otherwise.

P. Paolantonio, C. Dromain, *Imaging of Small Bowel, Colon and Rectum*,   67
A-Z Notes in Radiological Practice and Reporting,
DOI 10.1007/978-88-470-5489-9_7, © Springer-Verlag Italia 2014

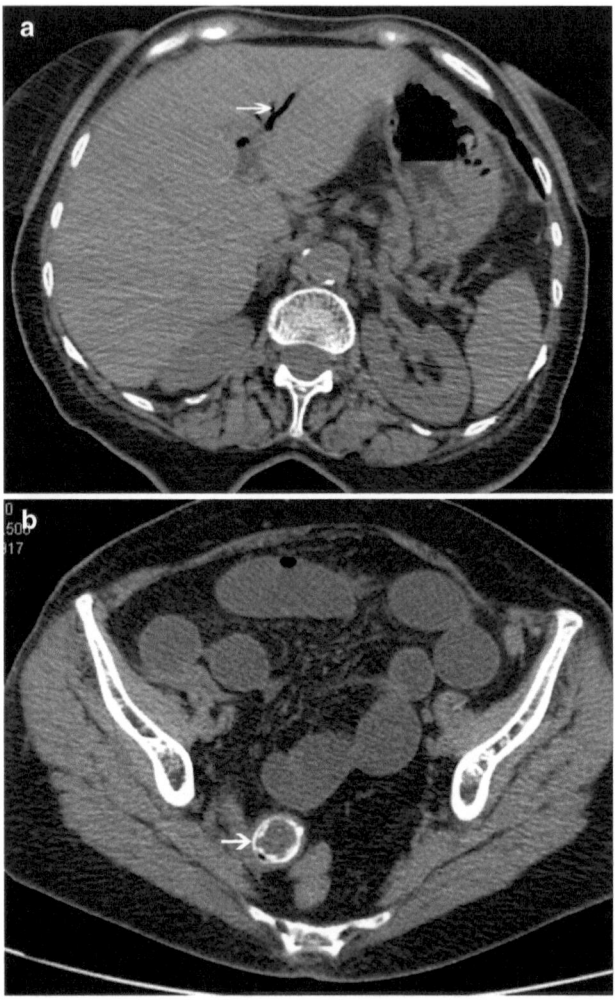

Fig. 1 CT images in a patient suffering with gallstone ileus. In (**a**) gas in the biliary duct is clearly visible (*arrow*); in (**b**) a calcified gallstone is visible in a pelvic small bowel loop with dilatation of upstream loops

- Pathogenesis is due to intestinal wall alteration permitting passage of air into venules. The intestinal ischemia is the most common cause of gas in the portal venous system. However other possible causes are represented by ulceration of gastric or duodenal wall, iatrogenic air distension of the gastrointestinal system (ERCP, colonoscopy), or intra-abdominal sepsis (gas from septicemia in branches of mesenteric veins).
- CT imaging is able to distinguish small amount of gas into tubular areas in the liver periphery as well as in portal and mesenteric veins. Main differential diagnosis is with pneumobilia (air located centrally in the liver within the bile ducts at the hilus and mainly in the left liver lobe).

Gastrografin®

- *Gastrografin* is the brand name of an iodinated oral contrast medium (diatrizoic acid) with high osmolarity administered orally or by enema to image the gastrointestinal system in patients with contraindications for barium sulfate. Thanks to its high osmolarity, it shows cathartic properties and it was proposed as tagging agent for fluid residual stool in the colon prior to virtual colonoscopy.

Giardiasis

- Giardiasis is a parasitic infection due to overgrowth of commensal parasite (Giardia lamblia) occurring in predisposed subject (altered immune mechanism). At histology giardiasis presents with blunted villi and cellular infiltrate of lamina propria and may be confused with celiac disease. Clinical feature widely ranges from symptomatic to severe diarrhea.

Infection is commonly located in the duodenum and jejunum with thickened and distorted fold with normal ileum. Diagnosis is based on detection of Giardia lamblia cyst in formed feces or trophozoites in diarrheal stools.

GIST

- Gastrointestinal stromal tumors (GISTs) are the most common mesenchymal tumor that arises in the muscularis propria layer of the bowel wall. They are well known to originate from precursors of interstitial cell of Cajal. KIT (CD117, a tyrosine kinase growth factor receptor) is usually positive (95 %). These tumors are occurring frequently in the stomach (60 %), small bowel (30 %), colon and rectum (5 %), and esophagus (<5 %) and few tumors are arising at the omentum, mesentery, and retroperitoneum.
- Endoscopic ultrasound and CT are the most widely used imaging modalities. MRI could be useful in staging anorectal disease, whereas FDG PET has been shown to be useful to assess early response to treatment.
- Radiologic features of GISTs vary depending on tumor size and organ of origin. They most commonly have an exophytic growth pattern and manifest as dominant masses outside the organ of origin. The typical imaging findings of GISTs are well-defined submucosal tumor with intact overlying mucosa. Intratumoral necrosis, hemorrhage, and perforation could be seen with tumor growing. On contrast-enhanced CT scan, small tumor shows homogeneous enhancement and large tumors show heterogeneous enhancement due to internal hemorrhage and necrosis (Fig. 2). GIST can cause variable complications, such as gastrointestinal hemorrhage, obstruction, torsion, intussusception, and rupture with hemoperitoneum. The imaging features of these tumors are usually not

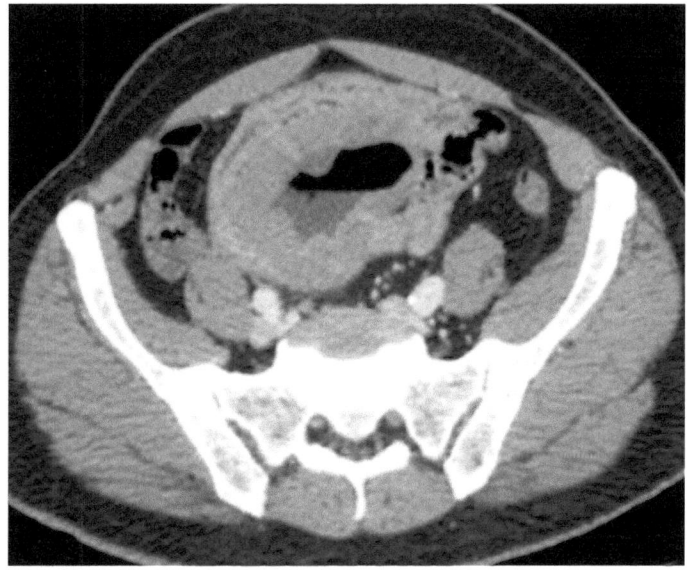

Fig. 2 Small bowel GIST. Axial contrast-enhanced CT image shows a large mass developing from the small bowel with intratumoral necrosis

characteristic, so the radiologic differential diagnosis is sometimes very difficult. The differential diagnoses of GIST are other submucosal tumors such as carcinoid tumor, neurogenic tumor, metastasis, inflammatory fibroid polyp, ectopic pancreas, or polypoid type of adenocarcinoma.

- Most of GISTs (60–70 %) are benign. The assessment of malignancy is based on tumor size, mitotic index, and spread outside the gastrointestinal tract. GISTs with high mitotic activity (>5 mitoses per high power field) are considered high grade and demonstrate aggressive behavior. Small bowel GISTs appear to follow a more aggressive course, compared to gastric tumors of the same size. CT prediction of malignancy is size >5 cm, irregular margins, local invasion, central necrosis or hemorrhage, exophytic growth pattern, and mesenteric infiltration, whereas the degree of enhancement is not correlated with risks of malignancy. The main sites of metastases are the liver and the peritoneum, often large, multiple, and hypervascularized with central necrosis and hemorrhage. GISTs rarely metastasize to the mediastinum, bone, lung, or subcutaneous sites

- CT is the modality of choice for follow-up. The timing must be adapted to the risk of malignancy: CT every 6 months for 3 years and then annually for 2 years in high-risk patients, CT at 9 months and then annually in intermediate risk, and CT at 1 year in low-risk patients.
- Imatinib mesylate, an orally administered competitive inhibitor of tyrosine kinases, is the treatment of choice of metastatic or inoperable patient. Choi criteria have been shown to be more accurate than criteria based on size measurement to assess response to treatment. A response is defined as a 10 % decrease in unidimensional tumor size or a 15 % decrease in tumor density on contrast-enhanced CT.

Suggested Reading

Goussous N, Eiken PW, Bannon MP, Zielinski MD (2013) Enhancement of a small bowel obstruction model using the gastrografin® challenge test. J Gastrointest Surg 17(1):110–117

Heye T, Bernhard M, Mehrabi A, Kauczor HU, Hosch W (2012) Portomesenteric venous gas: is gas distribution linked to etiology and outcome? Eur J Radiol 81(12):3862–3869

Hong X, Choi H, Loyer EM, Benjamin RS, Trent JC, Charnsangavej C (2006a) Gastrointestinal stromal tumor: role of CT in diagnosis and in response evaluation and surveillance after treatment with imatinib. Radiographics 26(2):481–495

Hong X, Choi H, Loyer EM, Benjamin RS, Trent JC, Charnsangavej C (2006b) Gastrointestinal stromal tumor: role of CT in diagnosis and in response evaluation and surveillance after treatment with imatinib. Radiographics 26(2):481–495, Review

Lassandro F, Romano S, Ragozzino A, Rossi G, Valente T, Ferrara I, Romano L, Grassi R (2005) Role of helical CT in diagnosis of gallstone ileus and related conditions. AJR 185:1159–1165

Lau S, Tam KF, Cam CK, Lui CY, Siu CW, Lam HS, Malk KL (2004) Imaging of gastrointestinal stromal tumor (GIST). Clin Radiol 59(6):487–498, Review

Orchard J, Petorack V (1995) Abnormal CT findings in patient with giardiasis. Digest Dis Sci 40(2):346–348

Rajendra R, Pollack SM, Jones RL (2013) Management of gastrointestinal stromal tumors. Future Oncol 9(2):193–206

H

Hartmann's Procedure

- Hartmann's procedure is a surgical resection of the rectosigmoid colon with closure of the rectal stump and formation of an end colostomy. It was used to treat colon cancer or diverticulitis. Currently its use is limited to emergency surgery when immediate anastomosis is not possible, or more rarely it is used palliative in patients with colorectal tumors.

Henoch–Schonlein Purpura

- Henoch–Schonlein purpura is the most common systemic acute small vessel vasculitis in children and young adults consisting in deposition of IgA-dominant immune complex in venules, capillaries, and arterioles. Most common clinical manifestations are purpuric skin rash, colicky abdominal pain and GI bleeding (gastrointestinal manifestation may anticipate cutaneous rash), microscopic hematuria and proteinuria, and arthralgia of large joints.

P. Paolantonio, C. Dromain, *Imaging of Small Bowel, Colon and Rectum*, 75
A-Z Notes in Radiological Practice and Reporting,
DOI 10.1007/978-88-470-5489-9_8, © Springer-Verlag Italia 2014

- At imaging gastrointestinal manifestation consists in multifocal bowel wall thickening (due to intramural hemorrhage and edema).

Hernia

- Hernia represents a common cause of small bowel obstruction. A main categorization divides hernia in two groups: internal and external hernia.
- *External hernia* consists in the bowel extending outside of the abdominal cavity and it is the most common hernia. Considering the site of herniation, we distinguish different types of external hernia:

Ventral

- *Postoperative hernia*
- *Trocar site hernia*
- *Umbilical hernia*
- *Epigastric hernia*
- *Spigelian hernia* (acquired ventrolateral hernia through a defect of aponeurosis between the rectum muscle of the abdomen)

Diaphragm

- *Morgagni and Bochdalek hernias*

Groin

- *Inguinal hernia*
  - *Direct* (medial to inferior epigastric vessels) containing bowel, mesenteric fat, and vessels
  - *Indirect* (lateral to inferior epigastric vessels originating at the deep inguinal ring)

- *Femoral hernia* (medial to femoral vein within femoral canal), with high risk of incarceration
- *Richter hernia* (entrapment of antimesenteric border of the bowel in hernia orifices, more common in femoral hernia and trocar site hernia)
- *Internal hernia* consists in herniation of the bowel through a developmental or surgical created defect of the peritoneum, omentum, mesenteric, or adhesive band. Different types of internal hernia are possible: *paraduodenal hernia*, *lesser sac hernia*, *and iatrogenic internal hernia*
- *Paraduodenal hernia*: through a congenital defect in the descending mesocolon (left side) or through mesentericoparietal fossa (right side); at CT an encapsulated bowel loop is detectable in abnormal position displacing anterolaterally the inferior mesenteric vein or anteriorly the right colic vein, respectively.
- *Lesser sac hernia*: through the foramen of Winslow (retrogastric hernia).
- *Iatrogenic internal hernia* (transmesenteric hernia): herniation through an iatrogenic fenestration of the mesocolon (central displacement of the colon).

Hirschsprung Disease

- Aganglionic megacolon or Hirschsprung disease is a congenital absence of parasympathetic ganglia in Meissner and Auerbach plexus leading to relaxation failure of the aganglionic segment.

Hyperplasia, Lymphoid

- Lymphoid hyperplasia (hyperplastic lymph follicles in lamina propria) represents a normal variant of the terminal ileum appearance in children and young adult or a self-limiting inflammatory/infective/allergic process.

- In adults, it may be associated with immunoglobulin deficiency.

Suggested Reading

Ha HK, Lee SH, Rha SE, Kim JH, Byun JY, Lim HY, Chung JW, Kim JG, Kim PN, Lee MG, Auh YH (2000) Radiologic features of vasculitis involving the gastrointestinal tract. Radiographics 20:779–794

Jamieson DH, Shipman PJ, Israel DM, Jacobson K (2003) Comparison of multidetector CT and barium studies of the small bowel: inflammatory bowel disease in children. AJR 180:1211–1216

Zarvan NP, Lee FT, Yandow DR, Unger JS (1995) Abdominal hernias: CT findings. AJR 164(1):391–1395

Ileocecal Valve Abnormalities

- Ileocecal valve is a papillose structure with physiologic sphincter muscle.
  It may have variable morphology (from a thin or thick labial structure to rounded morphology).
- *Lipomatosis* is a common abnormality of the ileocecal valve more frequent in women >40 years old. Several abnormalities may affect the ileocecal valve such as *lymphoid hyperplasia*, inflammatory process (Crohn's disease, ulcerative colitis, parasitic infections), intussusception, and neoplasm.
- Neoplasms of the ileocecal valve are represented by lipoma, adenomatous or villous polyp, carcinoid tumor, adenocarcinoma, and lymphoma (often involving the terminal ileum).

P. Paolantonio, C. Dromain, *Imaging of Small Bowel, Colon and Rectum*, 79
A-Z Notes in Radiological Practice and Reporting,
DOI 10.1007/978-88-470-5489-9_9, © Springer-Verlag Italia 2014

Ileus

- The term ileus refers to inability of the bowel to push fluid along with intestinal stasis. The term ileus itself does not distinguish between the mechanisms of the stasis (mechanical/nonmechanical causes). For mechanical ileus *see Bowel obstruction*. Terms *nonmechanical ileus*, *adynamic ileus*, and *nonobstructive ileus* are synonyms referring to intestinal stasis without a mechanical origin.
- Possible causes of adynamic ileus in adults are represented by:
  - *Postoperative ileus* (usually resolving in 4th postoperative day)
  - *Visceral pain* (obstructing ureteral stone, common bile duct stone, twisted ovarian cyst, blunt abdominal or chest trauma)
  - *Intra-abdominal inflammation/infection*: peritonitis, appendicitis, cholecystitis, pancreatitis, salpingitis, abdominal abscess, and ischemic bowel disease
  - Anticholinergic drugs
  - Neuromuscular and metabolic disorders: diabetes, hypothyroidism, uremia, hypokalemia, amyloidosis, myotonic dystrophy, CNS trauma, and paraplegia
  - *Systemic disease*: Septic and hypovolemic shock
  - *Retroperitoneal disease*: Hemorrhage and abscess
- Ileus presents with mild dilated small bowel loops *without transition zone*; after oral iodinated contrast medium administration, a delayed but free passage of contrast material can be detected.
- *Localized ileus*: Isolated distended bowel loop ("sentinel loop") adjacent to acute inflammatory process (acute pancreatitis, cholecystitis, appendicitis, diverticulitis, ureteral colic).

Inflammatory Polyp

- Inflammatory polyps are nonneoplastic polyp of the colon occurring in patients suffering with inflammatory bowel disease.

Infliximab®

- Infliximab is the brand name of the most common drug used in biologic therapy of inflammatory bowel disease as well as in many other autoimmune diseases.
- Infliximab is an anti-TNF alpha antibody that allows a down-regulation of inflammation leading to remission of active disease with excellent response of fistulas. Infliximab therapy presents also many side and adverse effects due to a certain degree of immunodepression induced. Moreover quick changes of inflammatory modification of bowel wall may evolve in intramural fibrosis and bowel lumen reduction with worsening of intestinal stricture in Crohn's disease patients. Therefore infliximab therapy is not indicated in patients with ongoing infectious disease and in case of intestinal strictures.

Insulinoma

- An insulinoma is an insulin-producing pancreatic NET and represents the most common pancreatic endocrine tumor that is derived from beta cells. This is a benign tumor in more than 90 % of cases.

- The classical clinical presentation is the Whipple triad associating starvation attack, hypoglycemia after fasting, and relief by i.v. dextrose.
- The diagnosis is usually made biochemically with low blood glucose and elevated insulin, proinsulin, and C-peptide levels. An increased level of chromogranin A is also a common marker of neuroendocrine tumors.
- The endo-ultrasonography is the imaging modality of choice for the detection of the tumor that is most often of small size. Moreover it allows the realization of a fine needle aspiration or microbiopsy for the histopathological diagnosis.
- CT examination requires the acquisition of images during the late arterial phase (30 s after the initiation of contrast administration) as well as a portal venous phase. Insulinoma is most often solitary, located in the body and tail localization, with small size <1.5 cm, and typically hypervascularized at the arterial phase. A ringlike enhancement has been described to be very suggestive of the diagnostic of insulinoma.
- On MRI, the tumor is often hyperintense on T2-weighted images, hypointense on fat-suppressed T1-weighted images, and hyperintense on the arterial phase. However the contrast to lesion is most often higher on unenhanced T1-weighted images than on arterial phase due to the high contrast enhancement of the normal pancreatic parenchyma.
- Somatostatin receptor imaging (using a scintigraphy or a PET technique) has a limited sensitivity in insulinomas. However it is less sensitive for the detection of insulinoma than for the other types of NETs (see Octreoscan).

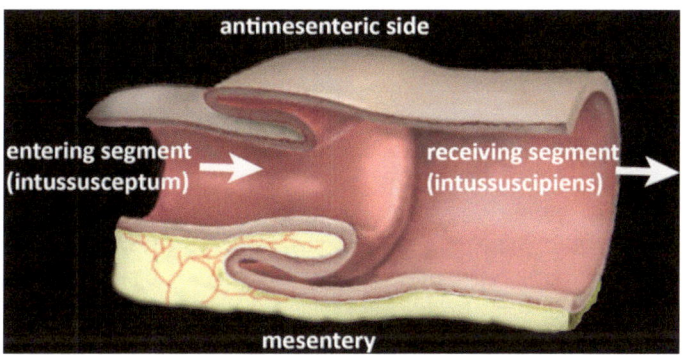

Fig. 1 Graphic describes the intestinal intussusception with a proximal intestinal segment (intussusceptum) prolapsing into a distal segment (intussuscipiens) following the peristaltic direction (*arrow*). Therefore at the site of intussusception, CT and MR imaging easily detect a multilayered structure composed by concentric layers: intussuscipiens bowel wall, folded intussuscipiens bowel wall, and intussusceptum bowel wall giving the overall image of a target with inner narrowed bowel lumen. Moreover on the mesenteric border, mesenteric fat can be detected between intussuscipiens and intussusceptum bowel wall

Intussusception

- Intestinal intussusception represents a cause of intestinal obstruction due to the invagination of an intestinal segment into another segment similar to the way of a collapsible telescope slid into one other. The part that prolapses into the other is called intussusceptum, while the part that receives is called intussuscipiens (Fig. 1).

- Intestinal intussusception may involve small bowel segments only (ileoileal intussusception) or terminal ileum and colon (ileocolic intussusception).
- Pathogenesis of intussusception regards the intestinal peristalsis that pulls a proximal segment into a distal segment. This happens more frequently if a pedunculated mass is present since the mass is easily pulled by peristalsis sliding the site of implants into the intussuscipiens segment. In patients affected by celiac disease or other intestinal disease, diffuse intestinal atony may lead to transient intussusception without the presence of intestinal mass and spontaneously resolving.
- At CT imaging intestinal intussusception is easily diagnosed, thanks to CT when an intestinal obstruction is seen with a layered appearance of the bowel at the transition zone with the so-called "bowel in the bowel" feature. The presence of mesenteric fat and vessels inner the intussusceptions bowel wall and outer respect the intussuscepted bowel wall an overall target appearance is a clue sign for intestinal intussusception. In details at CT multiple concentric ring appearance can be recognized in case of intussusception due to the presence of 3 concentric cylindrical structures. The central cylinder is the intestinal lumen plus wall of intussusceptum, the middle cylinder is the crescent of mesenteric fat, and the outer cylinder is the returning intussusceptum wall plus intussuscipiens wall.

Ischiorectal Fossa

- Ischiorectal fossa (or ischioanal fossa) is a fat-filled symmetric space located lateral to the anal canal and inferior to the levator ani muscle. Ischiorectal fossa represents the space of diffusion of transsphincteric, suprasphincteric, and extrasphincteric fistulas, while intersphincteric fistulas will never have an ischiorectal fossa involvement.

Suggested Reading

Caramella C, Dromain C, De Baere T, Boulet B, Schlumberger M, Ducreux M, Baudin E (2010) Endocrine pancreatic tumours: which are the most useful MRI sequences. Eur Radiol 20(11):2618–2627

Furukawa A, Yamasaki M, Furuichi K, Yokoyama K, Nagata T, Takahashi M, Murata K, Sakamoto T (2001) Helical CT in the diagnosis of small bowel obstruction. Radiographics 21:341–355

Kim YH, Blake MA, Harisinghani MG, Archer-Arroyo K, Hahn PF, Pitman MB, Mueller PR (2006) Adult intestinal intussusception: CT appearances and identification of a causative lead point. Radiographics 26:733–744

Seckl MJ, Mulholland PJ, Bishop AE, Teale JD, Hales CN, Glaser M et al (1999) Hypoglycemia due to an insulin-secreting small-cell carcinoma of the cervix. N Engl J Med 341(10):733–736

J

Jejunization of Ileum

- Jejunization of ileum is defined as an increased number of ileal folds (>3 folds/in.) leading to an appearance of the ileal loops similar to the jejunal loop. Jejunal loops are located in the upper left abdominal quadrant, while ileal loops are distributed in the other abdominal quadrants. It is possible to localize jejunal loops by drawing an imaginary line on coronal images from the gallbladder to the superior aspect of the left iliac bone. Jejunal loops are located above this line. Ileal jejunization is one of the imaging findings suggesting celiac disease.
- Ileal jejunization is one of the imaging findings suggesting celiac disease.

Juvenile Polyposis

- Juvenile polyposis is a syndrome characterized by the appearance of multiple polyps in the gastrointestinal tract in children, adolescents, young adults, and adults. Polyps are

P. Paolantonio, C. Dromain, *Imaging of Small Bowel, Colon and Rectum*,   87
A-Z Notes in Radiological Practice and Reporting,
DOI 10.1007/978-88-470-5489-9_10, © Springer-Verlag Italia 2014

nonneoplastic hamartomatous polyp. Commonly polyps are located in the colon and rectum. A solitary juvenile polyp occurs usually in the rectum and presents rectal bleeding.

Suggested Reading

Kopacova M, Tachei I, Reichrt S, Kopac BJ (2009) Peutz-Jeghers syndrome: diagnostic and therapeutic approach. World J Gastroenterol 15(43):5397–5408

Paolantonio P, Tomei E, Rengo M, Ferrari R, Lucchesi P, Laghi A (2007) Adult celiac disease: MRI findings. Abdom Imaging 32(4):433–440, Review

K

No Lemma

P. Paolantonio, C. Dromain, *Imaging of Small Bowel, Colon and Rectum*, 89
A-Z Notes in Radiological Practice and Reporting,
DOI 10.1007/978-88-470-5489-9_11, © Springer-Verlag Italia 2014

L

Levator Ani Muscle

- The levator ani muscle is a broad thin muscle of the pelvis; it supports pelvic viscera and structures that pass it through. The levator ani muscle in conjunction with the coccygeal muscle forms the pelvic diaphragm.
- The levator ani muscle is divided into three parts: the ileococcygeal muscle, pubococcygeal, and puborectal muscle.
- The contraction of all components of levator ani muscle realizes the rising up of the pelvic floor, and at the same time, thanks to the action of puborectal muscle, the anorectal junction is pushed anteriorly with reduction of anorectal angle.
- The relaxation of levator ani muscle leads to the opening of anorectal angle. Therefore the action of levator ani muscle and the specific action of one of its branches (puborectal muscle) play an important role in defecation and fecal continence as well as in pelvic floor disease such as *rectal prolapse, descending perineum syndrome, obstructed defecation syndrome, and abdominopelvic incoordination.*

- The levator ani muscle syndrome is characterized by episodical rectal pain (*proctalgia fugax*) due to spasm of the levator ani muscle.
- The levator ani muscle is also an important anatomical landmark in categorization of perianal fistula particularly in the definition of suprasphincteric and extrasphincteric fistulas in which the levator ani muscle is involved in the fistulous tract.
- MRI using phased-array coil, high magnetic field strength (1.5 T magnet) acquiring high spatial resolution TSE T2-weighted images on coronal and axial planes is the best imaging method to imagine the levator ani muscle from a morphologic point of view.
- MR defecography is used to investigate functionality of the levator ani muscle as well as the defecation function.

Lymphoma, GI Tract

- Gastric and duodenal lymphomas are most often B-cell non-Hodgkin's lymphoma (MNHL). Lymphomas may occur as a primary gastric lesion or as part of a disseminated disease. The primary location of MNHL in the stomach accounts for less than 5 % of malignant gastric tumors. However the stomach is the most common extranodal site of primary lymphomas.
- Symptoms include epigastric pain, early satiety, fatigue, and weight loss. These lymphomas are difficult to differentiate from gastric adenocarcinoma. However differentiating poor gastric lymphoma from adenocarcinoma is essential because the prognosis and modalities of treatment differ significantly.
- The main imaging feature of MNHL is thickening of the gastric wall greater than 10 mm interesting most or the entire stomach circumference. However, intraluminal fungating lesion, polypoid lesion, and ulcers have been described.

Persistent stomach distension capacity and the lack of appearance of the rigid wall, despite a significant thickening, are characteristics highly suggestive of lymphoma. This finding allows differentiating the lymphoma from a linitis plastica. The presence of a cleft within the thickened gastric wall and the presence of nodes of both sides of mesenteric vessels are also suggestive of lymphoma. Radiologic findings are present in about 69 % of gastric lymphomas. So a normal CT does not exclude the diagnosis of lymphoma.

- The characteristics of lymphoma located in the duodenum, the jejunum, and the ileum are similar to those of gastric lymphoma (Fig. 1). However, tortuous and pseudoaneurysmal forms have been described. Peritumoral lymph nodes are often voluminous.

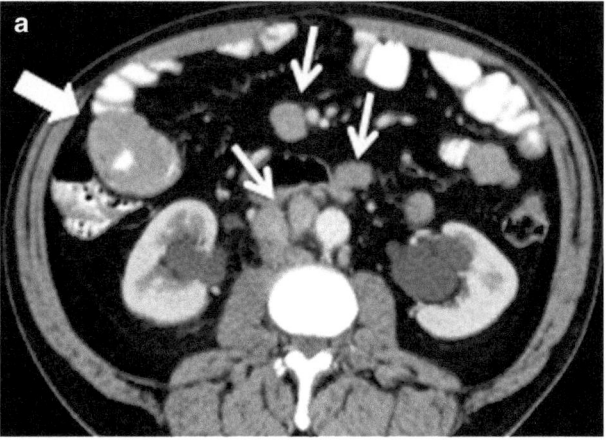

Fig. 1 Non-Hodgkin's lymphoma of the small bowel. Axial contrast-enhanced CT image (**a**) shows an important thickening of the ileal wall without obstruction (*large arrow*). Associated lymph nodes in the mesentery and the retroperitoneum (*arrows*) also well depicted on FDG PET image (**b**) are suggestive of lymphoma

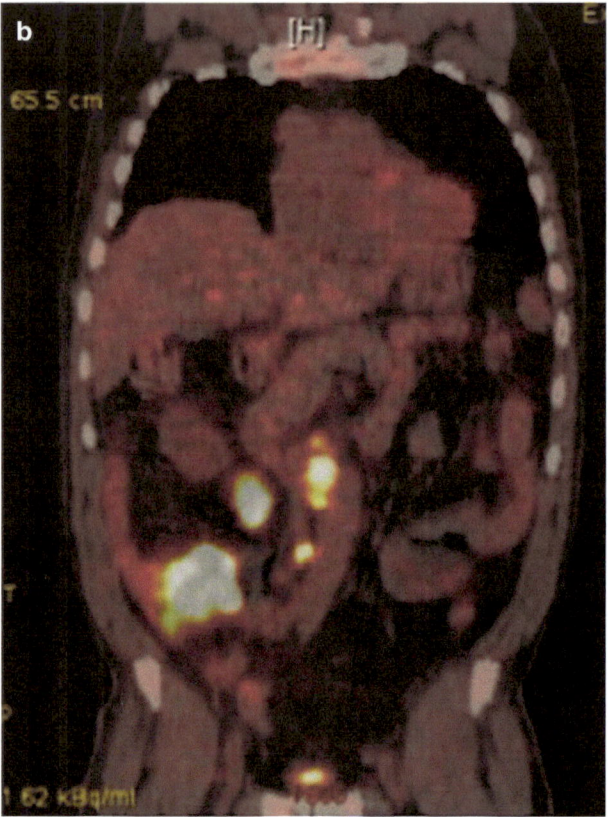

Fig. 1 (continued)

- The diagnosis is made by biopsy at the time of endoscopy. Endoscopic findings include solitary ulcers, thickened gastric folds, mass lesions, and nodules. CT examination is complementary to endoscopy to appreciate the extent of the lesion in and outside of the gastric wall and for the staging at distance.
- FDG PET could be also useful to assess the response to treatment.

Lipodystrophy, Mesenteric

• Mesenteric lipodystrophy (also known as chronic fibrosing mesenteritis, mesenteric panniculitis, liposclerotic mesenteritis) is a benign disorder of unknown etiology characterized by fibrofatty thickening of small bowel mesentery. Mesenteric panniculitis presents at CT as mesenteric fat thickening with interspersed soft tissue density (fibrous tissue) along the mesentery with multiple enlarged (<1 cm small axis) mesenteric lymph nodes that are frequently associated. Possible differential diagnosis is represented by mesenteric lymphoma and liposarcoma of the mesentery.

Lipoma, GI Tract

• Gastrointestinal lipoma is a benign submucosal tumor composed of mature adipose tissue most common in the colon (cecum and ascending colon) but often located at the level of duodenum and ileum. It can be asymptomatic or leading to crampy pain. At CT imaging, it is easily diagnosed presenting as a well-circumscribed submucosal fatty mass with uniform density.

Suggested Reading

Ghai S, Pattison J, Ghai S, O'Malley ME, Khalili K, Stephens M (2007) Primary gastrointestinal lymphoma: spectrum of imaging findings with pathologic correlation. Radiographics 27(5):1372–88

Laghi A, Iafrate F, Paolantonio P, Iannaccone R, Baeli I, Ferrari R, Catalano C, Passariello R (2002) Magnetic Resonance Imaging of the anal canal using high resolution sequences and phased array coil: visualization of anal sphincter complex. Radiol Med 103(4):353–9

Mason R, Bristol JB, Petersen V, Lyburn ID (2010) Education and imaging. Gastrointestinal: lipoma induced intussusception of the transverse colon. J Gastroenterol Hepatol 25(6):1177

Masselli G, Casciani E, Polettini E, Laghi F, Gualdi G (2013) Magnetic resonance imaging of small bowel neoplasms. Cancer Imaging 13:92–9

M

Malabsorption

- Malabsorption is defined as deficient absorption of any essential food materials within the small bowel. It can be primary or secondary.
- Celiac disease is the most common cause of primary malabsorption. Possible origin of secondary malabsorption consisted in a wide spectrum of diseases: parasites infections (Giardia, etc.), inflammatory condition (enteritis viral, bacterial, fungal, chronic inflammatory bowel disease), mechanical defects (fistulas), neurologic disorder (functional diarrhea in diabetes), endocrine disease (Zollinger–Ellison syndrome), drugs (cathartics), systemic disease (scleroderma, lupus, polyarteritis, amyloidosis), lymphoma, benign and malignant bowel tumors, pancreatic disease (pancreatitis, pancreatectomy, cystic fibrosis, pancreatic cancer), and hepatobiliary disease (biliary obstruction, chronic liver disease).

P. Paolantonio, C. Dromain, *Imaging of Small Bowel, Colon and Rectum*,
A-Z Notes in Radiological Practice and Reporting,
DOI 10.1007/978-88-470-5489-9_13, © Springer-Verlag Italia 2014

MALT Lymphoma

- MALT lymphoma is a form of malignant B-cell non-Hodg-kin's lymphoma (MNHL) involving the mucosa-associated lymphoid tissue. It is associated with a *Helicobacter pylori* bacterial infection and chronic inflammation. This is a low-grade lymphoma that grows slowly and remains confined to one organ for a relatively long time.
- It accounts for only about 5 % of all non-Hodgkin's lympho-mas. The most commonly affected organ is the stomach. Most gastric MALT lymphomas arise in patients in whom gastros-copy shows nonspecific features such as inflammation, super-ficial erosions, or ulceration. That is why the most frequent problem in the diagnosis of gastric MALT lymphoma is its differentiation from *H. pylori*-associated gastritis.
- On CT imaging, the MALT lymphoma often appears as a thickening of the stomach wall that is focal and moderate. This finding highlighted the necessity to have a good disten-sion with water during CT examination.
- The diagnosis is made by biopsy at the time of endoscopy. Simultaneous tests for *H. pylori* are also done to detect the presence of this bacterium.
- MALT lymphomas remain localized in the majority of cases. However, 25–35 % of MALT lymphomas, more frequently among nongastric than gastric cases, present with dissemi-nated disease. Locoregional staging of gastric MALT lym-phoma is conducted by endoscopic ultrasonography and CT. An increasing depth of invasion of lymphoma through the stomach wall, depicted using endoscopic ultrasonography, has been reported to be closely correlated with decreasing responsiveness to *H. pylori* eradication treatment. Similarly, the involvement of the regional lymph nodes (which occurs in approximately 15–30 % of gastric MALT lymphomas) is

associated with considerably reduced response rates to either antibiotics or conventional treatment. The bone marrow is involved in this lymphoma in up to 15 % of cases, and less than 10 % of patients have distant lymph node involvement.

- Treatment is tailored to organ involvement and stage at presentation. Eradication of *Helicobacter pylori* using a triple anti-H. *pylori* regimen is standard therapy for all *Helicobacter pylori*-positive gastric MALT lymphomas. FDG PET could be useful to follow MALT lymphoma under treatment.

Meckel Diverticulum

- A Meckel diverticulum, a true congenital diverticulum, is a small bulge in the small intestine present at birth. It is a vestigial remnant of the omphalomesenteric duct.
- Meckel diverticulum is located in the distal ileum, usually within about 60–100 cm (2 ft) of the ileocecal valve. This *blind segment* or small pouch is about 3–6 cm long and may have a greater lumen diameter than that of the ileum. Heterotopic rests of the gastric mucosa and pancreatic tissue are seen in 60 and 6 % of cases, respectively.
- A memory aid is the rule of 2s: 2 % (of the population), 2 ft (from the ileocecal valve), 2 in. (in length), 2 % are symptomatic, 2 types of common ectopic tissue (gastric and pancreatic), 2 years is the most common age at clinical presentation, and 2 times *more boys are affected.* The majority of people afflicted with Meckel diverticulum are asymptomatic. If symptoms do occur, they typically appear before the age of 2.
- The most common presenting symptom is painless rectal bleeding such as melena-like black offensive stools, followed by intestinal obstruction, volvulus, and intussusception. Occasionally, Meckel diverticulitis may present with all the features of acute appendicitis.

- A technetium-99m (99mTc) pertechnetate scan, also called Meckel scan, is the investigation of choice to diagnose Meckel diverticula. This scan detects gastric mucosa since approximately 50 % of symptomatic Meckel diverticula have ectopic gastric or pancreatic cells contained within them; this is displayed as a spot on the scan distant from the stomach itself. This scan is highly accurate and noninvasive, with 95 % specificity and 85 % sensitivity.
- Computed tomography (CT scan) might be a useful tool to demonstrate a blind-ended and inflamed structure in the mid-abdominal cavity, which is not an appendix.

Megacolon

- Two clinical forms of megacolon are possible: aganglionic megacolon (see Hirschsprung disease) and *toxic megacolon.*
- *Toxic megacolon* is an acute transmural fulminant colitis with neurogenic loss of motor tone and rapid development of extensive colonic dilatation (>5.5 cm in transverse colon). Toxic megacolon represents commonly a complicating condition of ulcerative colitis; however, it can also be observed in patients with Crohn's disease, salmonellosis, pseudomembranous colitis, and ischemic colitis. Clinical features of toxic megacolon are represented by systemic toxicity and profuse bloody diarrhea with colonic ileus at X-rays (marked dilatation of transverse colon with air–fluid levels) and increasing caliber of the colon on serial radiographs).
- At CT toxic megacolon appears with distended colon with large amount of fluids and air, lack of colon or rectal obstruction, irregular nodular contour of thin colonic wall, and possible intramural air collection (pneumatosis).

Mesenteric Cyst

- Mesenteric or omental cyst can result as a sequelae of mesenteric of omental hematoma or abscess (thick wall, internal septa) and otherwise can be the manifestation of a duplication cyst (unilocular with thin wall). In differential diagnosis pancreatic pseudocyst and cystic lymphangioma should be considered as well.

Mesenteric Lymphadenitis

- Mesenteric lymphadenitis represents a clinical entity whose symptoms relate to benign inflammation of lymph nodes in the bowel mesentery caused commonly by Yersinia enterocolitica or viral infection affecting children and young adults presenting usually with vomiting and abdominal pain (diffuse or localized in the right lower quadrant); diarrhea may be also present.
- Enlarged lymph nodes are usually in the small bowel mesentery but also anteriorly to the right psoas muscle. Sometimes mild thickening of the ileal or colonic wall can be evident. Visualization of the entire normal appendix is necessary to differentiate mesenteric lymphadenitis by acute appendicitis.

Mesenteric Venous Thrombosis

- Mesenteric venous thrombosis represents one of the mechanisms of acute mesenteric ischemia. Mesenteric venous thrombosis may result as a consequence of infection (sepsis, diverticulitis, appendicitis, peritonitis, abdominal abscess).

- Other possible causes of mesenteric venous thrombosis are represented by hypercoagulable status (antithrombin III deficiency, oral contraceptive therapy), abdominal trauma, or postoperative status. Mesenteric venous thrombosis may also be a consequence of intestinal volvulus or bowel obstruction.
- Symptoms may be subacute in early stage and evolve in severe abdominal pain with rebound tenderness, nausea, and vomiting. Hematemesis and hematochezia are present after bowel necrosis. Ileus and ascites may be also present.
- Contrast-enhanced CT is able to detect directly the thrombus within the mesenteric vein as a filling defect. In early stage of thrombosis, the vein is also increased in caliber, hyperattenuating at non-enhanced CT, and shows fat stranding of the surrounding mesenteric fat. SMV is involved more frequently with respect to IMV.

Mesorectum

- The mesorectum represents the enveloping mesentery of the rectum and is derived from the dorsal mesentery. The mesorectum contains fatty tissue, vessels, and lymphatics. It extends from the level of the peritoneal reflection down to the puborectalis muscle sling. The mesorectal fat is bounded by the mesorectal fascia.
- The mesorectum serves as a barrier to tumor growth and corresponds to the initial spread of tumor in rectal cancer. A major advancement in the treatment of rectal cancer was introduced in 1982 by the surgeon Richard John Heald. It consists in a total mesorectal excision which involves complete removal of the tumor along with the mesorectal tissue which contains the lymphatics and is associated with a drop in local recurrence rates from 40 to 11 %.
- The tumoral infiltration of the mesorectum is a key point of the staging of rectal tumors. When tumor grows through all

wall layers and extends into the mesorectum, the tumor is classified T3. Depending on the tumoral infiltration thickness of the mesorectum, the tumor is classified low T3 if this infiltration is less than one-third and strong T3 if it is greater than two-third of mesorectal thickness. MRI is the imaging modality of choice to analyze the mesorectum. On MRI the mesorectal fat has a high signal intensity on nonfat-suppressed T1- and T2-weighted images. MRI has a sensitivity of 82 % to detect perirectal tissue invasion.

Mesorectal Fascia

- The mesorectal fascia is the visceral layer of the endopelvic fascia that lines the rectum. It is a thin layer that maintains the integrity of the mesorectum. The mesorectal fascia is the resection plane in a total mesorectum excision.
- The endoscopic ultrasonography does not allow visualization of the mesorectal fascia, and MRI is currently the imaging method of choice to depict it. The mesorectal fascia is best seen on axial images as a fine line of low signal intensity. It appears as a fine low-signal-intensity structure enveloping the mesorectum (Fig. 1). The shortest distance from the tumor or lymph nodes to the mesorectal fascia is called the circumferential resection margin (CRM). It is the most powerful predictor for local recurrence.

MR Colonography

- MR colonography is a noninvasive radiation-free technique allowing a morphologic study of the colon; it was proposed to investigate non-acute colonic disease (colonic polyp, colon cancer, diverticular disease, and inflammatory bowel disease).

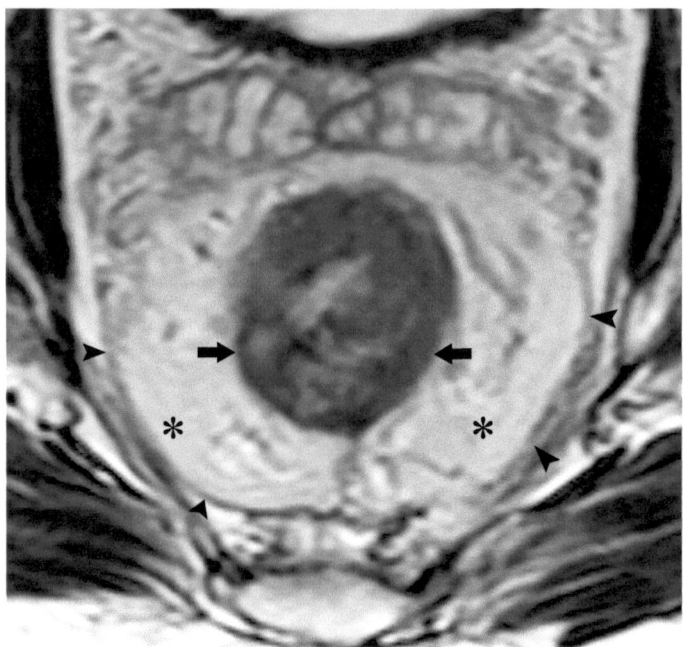

Fig. 1 MR T2-weighted image acquired on axial plane showing the meso-rectal fascia (*arrowheads*), mesorectal fat (*asterisk*) containing lymphatics and tiny blood vessels, and rectal wall (*arrows*)

- MR colonography is based on MR imaging of the abdomen performed after colonic cleansing and colonic distension by means of water enema. MR protocol sequences consisted in the acquisition of both fast T2-weighted or steady-state sequence and 3D GRE T1-weighted sequences acquired before and after i.v. administration of Gd-chelate. However, despite its great potential, MR colonography is not used routinely if not in a limited number of centers.

MR Defecography

- MR defecography is a noninvasive radiation-free imaging method used to study the morphology of pelvic floor as well as its function during defecation.
- MR defecography requires a short patient preparation with a rectal cleansing enema the day of the exam. Once in the MR suite, the rectum of the patient is filled by ultrasonographic gel by means of rectal tube. The exam is performed using phased-array coil for signal reception with patient in supine position using pads under patients to avoid damage to MR scanner due to leaking of sonographic gel.
- The study is composed by a morphologic assessment of pelvic floor by the acquisition of TSE T2-weighted images on axial, sagittal, and coronal planes and by a dynamic study of the pelvic floor performed acquiring a cine-FISP (fast imaging in the steady-state precession) sequence (one sagittal image passing through the pubic symphysis acquired continuously over time for 40 s). Dynamic study of the pelvic floor is acquired at rest, during contraction of the pelvic floor muscle, during straining, and finally during evacuation. Image analysis of dynamic study is aimed to assess qualitatively and quantitatively the behavior of the pelvic floor and pelvic organs in a dynamic manner. An important landmark to define the pelvic organ position is represented by the pubococcygeal line drawn from the inferior pubic symphysis to the last coccygeal articulation. The degree of prolapse of the pelvic organ is measured quantitatively from the pubococcygeal line. The rectal prolapse is measured as the distance of the anorectal angle from the pubococcygeal line.
- MR defecography is indicated for the study of descending perineum syndrome, rectal prolapse, and abdominopelvic incoordination and in differential diagnosis of obstructed defecation syndrome giving important information to surgeon for an adequate treatment planning.

MR Enterography/Enteroclysis

- MR enterography and MR enteroclysis are MR dedicated studies of the small bowel performed after distending the small bowel using oral contrast agent (MR enterography) or water administration through a nasojejunal tube (RM enteroclysis). MR enterography is an easier and less time-consuming exam with respect to MR enteroclysis; however, MR enteroclysis achieves a reproducible distension of the entire small bowel even if a stricture is not present and therefore is more accurate in the identification of tiny bowel lesion without significant luminal obstruction.
- For MR enterography PEG or mannitol solution can be used as oral contrast agent at a dose of 1.5 l for adults and 10 ml/kg body weight in children. Oral assumption should be performed 20 min before patient positioning in the MR scanner to achieve distal ileum distension with 30 ml administered immediately before patient positioning to obtain distension of the duodenum and proximal jejunal loops. Prokinetic drug such as metoclopramide can be orally administered to enhance gastric emptying, and antispastic agent such as Buscopan or glucagon can be administered once the intestinal distension is optimally achieved to reduce motion artifact.
- MR protocol sequence is the same for both enterography and enteroclysis approach and is based on phased-array coil for signal reception and acquisition of fast T2-weighted sequence, FISP sequences, and Gd-chelate-enhanced T1-weighted sequence (dynamic administration is not necessary) acquired on axial and coronal planes. One of the major clinical indications for MR enterography/enteroclysis is represented by the diagnosis and follow-up of ileal Crohn's disease, thanks to the ability of MRI to detect bowel wall and mesentery inflammatory changes and to distinguish between bowel wall edema and fibrosis.

Mucocele, Appendix

- Mucocele of the appendix is a distension of the appendix with sterile mucus due to cystic dilatation of lumen secondary to obstruction by fecalith, foreign body, carcinoid, endometriosis, or adhesion. Other possible causes of mucocele are represented by mucosal hyperplasia or presence of mucinous cystoadenoma within the hyperplastic mucosa. A more rare condition leading to mucocele of the appendix is represented by the accumulation of thick mucus in patients with cystic fibrosis.
- Mucocele can be asymptomatic or leading to right lower quadrant abdominal pain (either acute or chronic) with palpable abdominal mass.
- At CT imaging mucocele presents with a round sharply defined paracecal mass with homogeneous near-water or soft tissue attenuation depending on amount of mucin.
- Complications of appendiceal mucocele are represented by rupture with pseudomyxoma peritonei, torsion with gangrene and hemorrhage, herniation in the cecum with intussusceptions, and bowel occlusion.

Suggested Reading

Arrivé L, El Mouhadi S, Masselli G, Gualdi G (2013) MR enterography versus MR enteroclysis. Radiology 266(2):688

Autenrieth DM, Baumgart DC (2012) Toxic megacolon. Inflamm Bowel Dis 18(3):584–591

Bello Báez A, Cavada A, Alventosa E, González C, Fernández Del Castillo M, Santana A, Vivancos JI, Pascual S, Rodríguez LE, Garrido MA, Fuentes J, Allende A, Domínguez Del Toro A (2008) Appendicular mucocele – multislice CT imaging. Rev Esp Enferm Dig 100(9): 592–593

Flusberg M, Sahni VA, Erturk SM, Mortele KJ (2011) Dynamic MR defecography: assessment of the usefulness of the defecation phase. AJR Am
J Roentgenol 196(4):394–399

Guettrot-Imbert G, Boyer L, Piette JC, Delèvaux I, André M, Aumaître O
(2012) Mesenteric panniculitis. Rev Med Interne 33(11):621–627

Iafrate F, Laghi A, Paolantonio P, Rengo M, Mercantini P, Ferri M, Ziparo
V, Passariello R (2006) Preoperative staging of rectal cancer with MR
Imaging: correlation with surgical and histopathologic findings.
Radiographics 26(3):701–714

Kämpf M, Adam P, Bares R, Brechtel K, Heuschmid M, Horger M (2012)
Imaging findings in complications of Meckel's Diverticulum: a rare differential diagnosis in acute abdomen. Rofo 184(9):765–768

Shaheen S, Guddati AK (2013) Secondary mucosa-associated lymphoid tissue (MALT) lymphoma of the colon. Med Oncol 30(2):502

Wong YC, Wu CH, Wang LJ, Chen HW, Lin BC, Huang CC (2013)
Mesenteric vascular occlusion: comparison of ancillary CT findings
between arterial and venous occlusions and independent CT findings
suggesting life-threatening events. Korean J Radiol 14(1):38–44

Zijta FM, Bipat S, Stoker J (2010) Magnetic resonance (MR) colonography
in the detection of colorectal lesions: a systematic review of prospective
studies. Eur Radiol 20(5):1031–1046

N

Neuroendocrine Tumor

- Neuroendocrine tumors (NETs) are a wide-ranging group of rare tumors that develop from neuroendocrine cells. The most common NETs arise from the gastrointestinal tract (including ileal and appendiceal tumor), lung, duodenum, and pancreas. Less often NET tumors can arise from the rectum, the stomach, the esophagus, and the larynx. NETs share common clinical features including hormone secretion, their possible association with an inherited syndrome, and a long-term natural history in a subgroup of well-differentiated endocrine carcinoma. The two main prognostic parameters in NET are pathological differentiation and histological grade defined, according to the values of the mitotic index and Ki67 index. NETs can be benign or malignant, but their histological features are not sufficiently predictive of malignant behavior: invasion of adjacent organs or structures or metastatic lesions are often required to formally establish malignancy.

P. Paolantonio, C. Dromain, *Imaging of Small Bowel, Colon and Rectum*,   109
A-Z Notes in Radiological Practice and Reporting,
DOI 10.1007/978-88-470-5489-9_14, © Springer-Verlag Italia 2014

- NET-related symptoms are due to hormonal secretion, i.e., Zollinger–Ellison syndrome in case of pancreatic gastrinomas, hypoglycemia in case of insulinas, and flush and diarrhea in case of serotonin secretion, or to tumor burden itself such as weight loss, asthenia, anorexia, bowel obstruction, and jaundice. Some tumors are found incidentally during imaging. Chromogranin A (CgA) is the most relevant biochemical marker for the diagnosis and prognosis of NETs.

- Imaging of well-differentiated endocrine carcinoma has several goals including detection of the primary, tumor staging, and the identification of tumors forming part of the spectrum of an inherited syndrome a subgroup of NET.

- Computed tomography (CT) scan is the reference technique for the initial evaluation and follow-up of NET-associated metastases, as it allows the exploration of the most frequent location of the primary tumors as well as metastatic sites (i.e., liver, abdominal and thoracic lymph nodes, peritoneum, lung, and bones). Acquisition techniques must be standardized and optimized, including acquisitions at the late arterial (30 s after the beginning of injection) and portal venous (70–90 s after the beginning of injection) phases. CT enteroclysis technique is performed in case of suspected ileal primary tumor (Fig. 1). The contribution of arterial acquisition increases sensitivity (20 % up) of the detection of pancreatic primary tumors and liver metastases. Indeed most of NETs are hypervascularized tumors with high contrast enhancement during the late arterial phase. CT scan is complementary to somatostatin receptor imaging, CT scan being more sensitive for the detection of lung, liver, and brain metastases and somatostatin receptor imaging for bones and mediastinum exploration.

- The contribution of magnetic resonance imaging (MRI) in regard to CT scan is important in the detection of NET liver metastases. MRI was reported to have a better sensitivity for

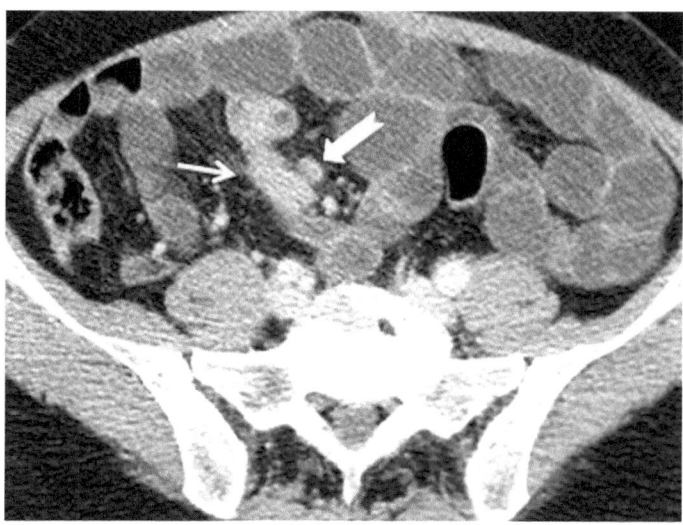

Fig. 1 Axial contrast-enhanced enteroclysis CT images shows a segmental enhancing thickening of the distal small bowel (arrow) associated with a mesenteric lymph node (large arrow) very suggestive of a primary neuroendocrine tumor

the detection of liver metastases in comparison with ultrasonography, CT scan, and SRS, comparable to the per-operatory ultrasonographic assessment but inferior to histological examination when performed on 3 mm thin slice sections. Diffusion-weighted sequence increases the sensitivity of MRI in NETs, particularly in hepatic miliary forms. Liver MRI is thus recommended to be performed in addition to CT scan in the initial morphologic assessment and before surgery.

- In patients with gastro-entero-pancreatic endodermal-derived ET, clinicians have taken advantage of somatostatin receptor imaging with radiolabeled octreotide (using either scintigraphy or PET imaging), a functional imaging modality for tumor staging. It allows visualization of the somatostatin receptors and especially subtype 2 which is expressed by the great majority of well-differentiated endocrine carcinoma should be considered as a complementary conventional imaging tool in patients with ET. Somatostatin receptor imaging is useful in pre-therapeutic assessment and follow-up. Moreover its positivity is suggestive of the neuroendocrine nature of a tumor and a good prognosis marker.

Suggested Reading

Dromain C, de Baere T, Lumbroso J, Caillet H, Laplanche A, Boige V, Ducreux M, Duvillard P, Elias D, Shlumberger M, Sigal R, Baudin E (2005) Detection of liver metastases from endocrine tumors: a prospective comparison of somatostatin receptor scintigraphy, computed tomography and magnetic resonance imaging. J Clin Orthod 23:70–78

Muniraj T, Vignesh S, Shetty S, Thiruvengadam S, Aslanian HR (2013) Pancreatic neuroendocrine tumors. Dis Mon 59(1):5–19

O

Obstructed Defecation Syndrome

- Obstructed defecation syndrome is a cause of constipation; symptoms include incomplete or unsuccessful attempts to evacuate, prolonged episodes on the toilet, rectal pain and tenesmus, digitations or perineal massage to aid defecation, and enema dependency. Fecal incontinence may be associated to gas or liquid stool, or urinary incontinence may be associated to the obstructed defecation syndrome (suggesting descending perineum syndrome). Obstructed defecation syndrome can be classified in different groups with different causes:

  - *Functional* (pelvic floor dyssynergia)
  - *Mechanical outlet obstruction* (mucosal rectal prolapse with intussusception and/or enterocele)
  - *Dissipation of force vector* (rectocele, descending perineum syndrome)

- Differential diagnosis among the mechanism of obstructed defecation syndrome which is crucial, leading to differences in patient management. MR defecography represents a morphologic and dynamic study of the pelvic floor that

P. Paolantonio, C. Dromain, *Imaging of Small Bowel, Colon and Rectum*,   113
A-Z Notes in Radiological Practice and Reporting,
DOI 10.1007/978-88-470-5489-9_15, © Springer-Verlag Italia 2014

allows a one-stop-shop examination in patients with obstructed defecation syndrome. MR defecography is able to study, without using ionizing radiation, the anterior pelvic floor compartment (bladder), as well as medium (uterus) and posterior compartment (rectum) combining morphologic information with functional information.

Octreoscan

- The octreoscan is the somatostatin receptor scintigraphy (SRS) using a radiolabeled somatostatin analog (^{111}In-octreotide or ^{111}In-pentetreotide) prior to scintigraphy with a large-field gamma camera. It visualizes the tumors with high expression of SST-2 receptors which are expressed by the great majority of well-differentiated endocrine carcinoma in both the primary neoplasm and the metastases. Its positivity is suggestive of the neuroendocrine nature of a tumor and a good prognosis marker. Moreover, this is a functional imaging modality complementary to morphologic imaging for well-differentiated NET staging, useful in pre-therapeutic assessment and follow-up. In conjunction with CT or MRI, octreoscan may be particularly helpful in identifying previously unsuspected extrahepatic and lymph node metastases. The specificity of octreoscan is high, but its sensitivity is variable depending on the size and the type of the tumor with a lower sensitivity in infracentimeteric tumors and in insulinomas. Across various types of NETs, the sensitivity of octreoscan is unaffected by vascularity or secretory activity of the neoplasms.
- In comparison with SRS negativity, SRS positivity was associated with longer overall survival and progression-free survival. SRS degree of positivity has been also reported to be a strong predictive factor of response to treatment with either

somatostatin analogs or internal irradiation with radioactive radiolabeled analogs. However, SRS is not relevant to characterize tumor progression, either spontaneous or under treatment.

Suggested Reading

Alexander HR, Fraker DL, Norton JA, Bartlett DL, Tio L, Benjamin SB, Doppman JL, Goebel SU, Serrano J, Gibril F, Jensen RT (1998) Prospective study of somatostatin receptor scintigraphy and its effect on operative outcome in patients with Zollinger-Ellison syndrome. Ann Surg 228(2):228–38

Muniraj T, Vignesh S, Shetty S, Thiruvengadam S, Aslanian HR (2013) Pancreatic neuroendocrine tumors. Dis Mon 59(1):5–19

Zbar AP (2013) Posterior pelvic floor disorders and obstructed defecation syndrome: Clinical and therapeutic approach. Abdom Imaging 38(5): 894–902

P

Parks Classification

- Parks classification is a widespread classification system for fistula in ano proposed by Parks in 1976. Parks described four different types of perianal fistula considering the fistulous tract with respect to the anal sphincter complex. Crucial landmarks for this classification are represented by the external anal sphincter and by the levator ani muscle. Four types of fistulas are described by Parks: intersphincteric, transphincteric, extrasphincteric, and suprasphincteric. Parks classification is very useful since different types of fistulas categorized using Parks methods require different surgical approach. Basically the intersphincteric fistula (i.e., the more easy and common fistula) can be treated with surgical fistulectomy, whereas other types of fistulas in whom the fistulous tract involves the external anal sphincter or the levator ani muscle should be treated with surgical drainage by means of seton positioning in order to avoid iatrogenic damage to sphincter complex and possible fecal incontinence.
- MRI of the pelvis is very useful in mapping noninvasively the fistulous tract and all possible distant abscess allowing an

P. Paolantonio, C. Dromain, *Imaging of Small Bowel, Colon and Rectum*, 117
A-Z Notes in Radiological Practice and Reporting,
DOI 10.1007/978-88-470-5489-9_16, © Springer-Verlag Italia 2014

accurate surgical planning and reducing the rate of fistula recurrence after surgery. However in many centers fistula in ano is imaged by endorectal ultrasound (using dedicated endorectal probe with 3D capabilities). Nevertheless MRI is strongly recommended in Crohn's disease patients presenting with anal fistula (complex fistulas) in diagnosis as well as in follow-up during medical treatment (infliximab therapy). In this last clinical setting as well as in complex fistulas, in recurrent fistulas, or in case of differential diagnosis between perianal abscess and mucinous tumor of the rectum and anal canal, the i.v. administration of Gd-chelates during MR exam may give additional information to conventional T2-weighted images study.

Pelvic Floor Dyssynergia

- Pelvic floor dyssynergia refers to a failure to the normal relaxation of pelvic floor during defecation, leading to obstructed defecation syndrome. MR defecography is able to detect the lack of relaxation of pelvic floor as well as the paradoxical contraction of puborectal muscle when the patient attempts to defecate, leading to the closening of anorectal angle with outlet mechanical pelvic obstruction. Digital examination and anorectal manometry are important tests; however, MR defecography is extremely important in the differential diagnosis with other causes of obstructed defecation syndrome. Therapy of pelvic floor dyssynergia is represented by biofeedback training. Some authors proposed the injection of botulinum toxin type A into the puborectal muscle in conjunction with biofeedback training.

Perforation, GI Tract

- Gastrointestinal perforation is a cause of acute abdomen.
- Gastrointestinal perforation is defined as a complete penetration of the wall of the stomach, small intestine, or large bowel resulting in intestinal contents flowing into the abdominal cavity. Perforation of the intestines results in the potential for bacterial contamination of the abdominal cavity with peritonitis. Perforation of the stomach can lead to a chemical peritonitis due to leaked gastric acid. Perforation anywhere along the gastrointestinal tract is a surgical emergency. Underlying causes include gastric ulcer, diverticulitis, appendicitis, gastrointestinal cancer, acute mesenteric ischemia, trauma, nonsteroidal anti-inflammatory drugs, and ingestion of corrosives. Perforation may also be iatrogenic during endoscopic procedures (ERCP, colonoscopy) or during abdominal surgery.
- CT scan can easily detect also small amount of peritoneal free air as indirect sign of perforation (Fig. 1). However the exact identification of perforation site is less easy. The direct sign of bowel wall defect is not always detectable. While some indirect findings can suggest the site of perforation such as perivisceral focal fat stranding, focal bowel wall thickening or the localized presence of gas bubble surrounding the bowel. The site of free air accumulation is not always associated with the site of perforation because, also in case of sigmoid perforation, air accumulates progressively in the subphrenic space progressively. On the other hand, the presence of air in the retroperitoneal space suggests an extraperitoneal site of perforation (right pararenal space for duodenal perforation).

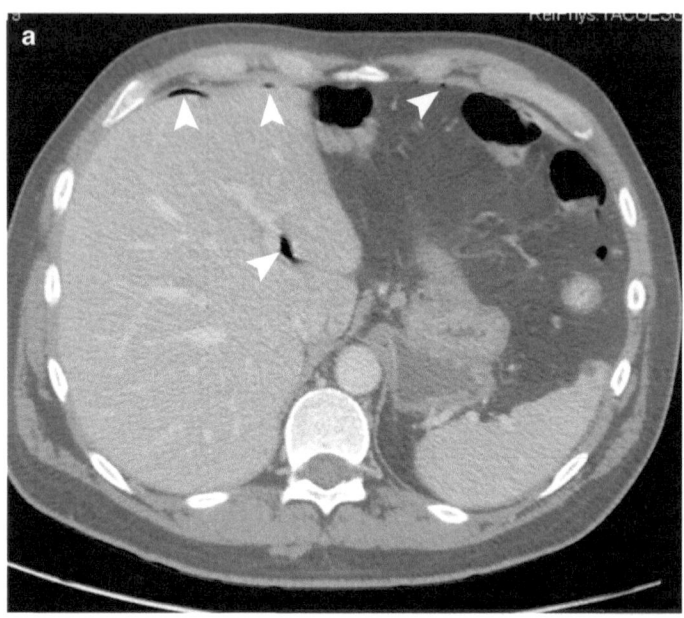

Fig. 1 (**a**) Shows small amounts of free intraperitoneal parahepatic air using lung windowing. In (**b** and **c**), a coronal MPR and axial pelvic scan are shown, respectively, showing sigmoid wall thickening with sign of diverticulitis (*asterisk*) and ileocolic fistula (*arrowhead*) and small extravisceral air pocket with associated ileus suggesting the sigmoid colon and complicated diverticulitis as site and cause of perforation, respectively

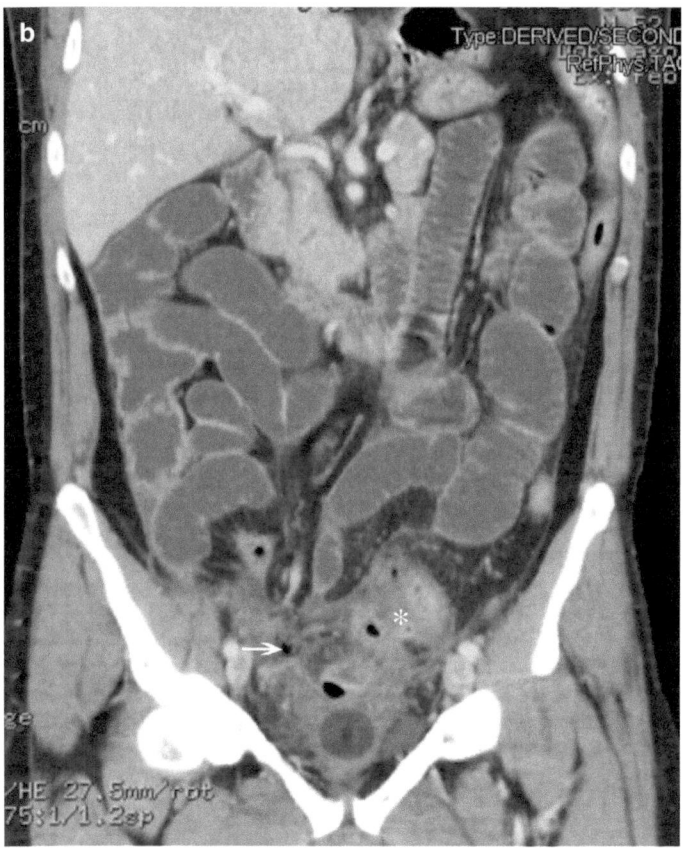

Fig. 1 (continued)

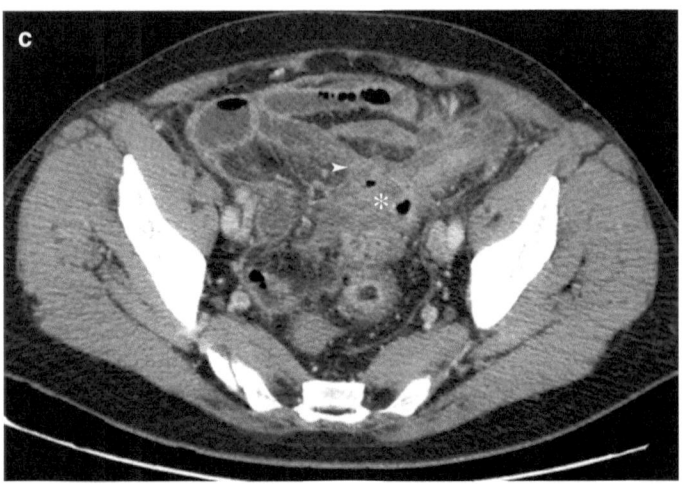

Fig. 1 (continued)

Peritonitis

- Peritonitis is an inflammation of the peritoneum; it may be localized or generalized, and it may result from infection (often due to perforation of the bowel or rupture of abdominal organ) or from a noninfectious process (leakage of sterile body fluids into peritoneum). However also noninfective peritonitis transforms into infective peritonitis over time. Sterile abdominal surgery can lead to a minimally localized or generalized noninfective auto-imitating peritonitis with associated dynamic ileus that may result sometimes in fibrotic peritoneal adhesion.

- More rare conditions are represented by spontaneous bacterial peritonitis (a peculiar form of peritonitis occurring in absence of obvious cause of contamination in patients with ascites) and tubercular peritonitis resulting from systemic TBC infections.
- A rare form of peritonitis is represented by sclerosing encapsulating peritonitis that represent an evolution of a simple peritoneal sclerosis in patients treated by means of long-term peritoneal dialysis.
- CT represents the imaging of choice to individuate the origin of peritonitis.

Pneumatosis Cystoides Intestinalis

- Pneumatosis cystoides intestinalis or cystic pneumatosis of the bowel (more frequently colonic cystic pneumatosis) is a rare condition characterized by multiple gas-filled cysts within the colon wall. Cystic pneumatosis of the colon has an uncertain origin, may be idiopathic or secondary to bacterial overgrowth, increased hydrogen gas production, and increased mucosal permeability and migration of gas into the bowel wall. Other mechanical iatrogenic causes are described such as colon insufflations during colonoscopy, barium enema, or virtual colonoscopy. Cystic pneumatosis may be associated also with lung disease or occurs in patients after organ transplantation. However cystic pneumatosis is characterized by a benign prognosis and can be incidental findings at CT imaging in patients with poor gastrointestinal symptoms. Diagnosis at CT colonography is easy; a differential diagnosis with other life-threatening cause of intestinal pneumatosis such as bowel infarction is essential for patient management.

Polyp

- Polyp is defined as a mass projecting into the lumen of a hollow viscus above the level of mucosa; usually polyp arises from mucosa; less frequently they may derive from submucosa (leiomyoma).
- Considering polyp morphology three main categories are described: sessile polyp, pedunculated polyp, and flat lesion (see carpet lesion).
- Polyps can be categorized at histology into two main categories: neoplastic (adenoma/carcinoma) and nonneoplastic (hamartoma/inflammatory).
- Neoplastic polyp of the colon (adenomatous polyp) is a precancerous lesion; a sequence adenoma to carcinoma on a long time interval (over 10-year time period) is recognized to be the origin of most part of colon–rectal carcinoma, while a small percentage of sporadic colonic carcinoma arises spontaneously without a previous detectable adenomatous polyp.
- Therefore a screening of colonic carcinoma is possible consisting in detecting and removing neoplastic polyps before their degeneration into colonic carcinoma. Neoplastic polyps (significant polyp) usually have considerable size (10 mm or more). Polyps smaller that 6 mm are usually nonneoplastic polyp.
- Considering CT colonography performances in terms of polyp detection, excellent results are reported for significant polyp (>10 mm size), while sensitivity and specificity decreases progressively for smaller-sized polyps especially for polyps <6 mm in maximum diameter. Due to the poor clinical meaning of polyps smaller than 6 mm and the false-negative and false-positive rate of CT colonography for these polyps, a consensus was achieved to avoid reporting polyp

smaller than 6 mm if their presence is uncertain on CT images.

- However a 5-year follow-up study is suggested for screening purpose after a negative CT colonoscopy instead of the 10-year follow-up applied for optical colonoscopy in the same clinical setting.

Polyposis

- Polyposis syndromes are defined as the presence of more than 100 polyps.
  Different polyposis syndromes are described with different transmission (hereditary/nonhereditary).
- Hereditary polyposis syndrome with autosomal dominant transmission is represented by familial adenomatous polyposis syndrome, Gardner syndrome, Peutz–Jeghers syndrome, and juvenile polyposis coli.
  Autosomal recessive hereditary mechanism is described for the Turcot syndrome.
- Nonhereditary polyposes are represented by Cronkhite–Canada syndrome and juvenile polyposis.
- Considering polyps histology in familial multiple polyposis, the Gardner and Turcot syndrome adenomatous polyps are founded.
- While hamartomatous polyps are described in Peutz–Jeghers syndrome (most in small bowel), Juvenile polyposis and Cronkhite–Canada syndrome.
- Moreover some polyposis look-alike condition exists, and they are represented by inflammatory polyposis, lymphoid hyperplasia, lymphoma, and cystic pneumatosis of the colon multiple bowel metastases (usually from melanoma).

Pseudopolyp

- Pseudopolyp is defined as a scattered island of inflamed edematous mucosa on a background of denuded mucosa. Pseudopolyps may occur in inflammatory bowel disease (pseudopolyposis of ulcerative colitis or cobblestoning of Crohn's disease).
- Post-inflammatory polyp is a filiform fingerlike projection of submucosa covered by mucosa on all sides following healing and regeneration of inflammatory disease (ulcerative colitis, ischemic or infectious bowel disease).

Pseudomembranous Colitis

- Pseudomembranous colitis is a nosocomial acute infectious colitis due to *Clostridium difficile* and its toxins (toxin A, enterotoxin; toxin B, cytotoxin).
- Predisposition factors are represented by antibiotic therapy (tetracycline, penicillin, ampicillin, amoxicillin, chloramphenicol, cephalosporins) or chemotherapeutic agents (methotrexate, fluorouracil) due to decrease of intestinal normal flora that usually opposed the proliferation of *Clostridium difficile*.
  Other predisposition factors are represented by abdominal surgery, renal transplantation, radiotherapy, prolonged hypotension, shock, uremia, colonic obstruction, debilitating disease (leukemia, advanced HIV infection), and immunosuppressive therapy.
- *Clostridium difficile* infection may be asymptomatic or, in a minority of cases, lead to antibiotic-associated colitis (without pseudomembranes) or pseudomembranous colitis, and in rare cases the so-called fulminant colitis is described (profuse

watery diarrhea, abdominal cramps, fever, leukocytosis, and less commonly dehydration, megacolon, hypoalbuminemia, and anasarca).

- Pseudomembranes are composed of exudate, leukocytes, fibrin, mucin, and sloughed necrotic epithelium held in columns by mucus. Pseudomembranes are located on partially denuded mucosa.
- At CT a circumferential, diffuse colonic wall thickening with target sign and accordion sign and colonic dilatation may be seen.
- Differential diagnosis should consider acute stage of ulcerative colitis, ischemic colitis, inflammatory colitis, and diverticulitis.
- Complications are represented by toxic megacolon and perforation with peritonitis.
- Diagnosis should be confirmed by means of stool assay for *Clostridium difficile* cytotoxin, stool culture (very sensitive but not available for 2 days), direct visualization of pseudomembrane (yellow plaques 2–10 mm of diameter adherent to rectosigmoid mucosa at optical colonoscopy).
- Therapy consists in discontinuation or suspended antibiotics, administration of vancomycin/metronidazole, attention fluid, and electrolyte balance.

Pseudosacculation, Intestinal

- Intestinal pseudosacculation can be observed in gastrointestinal manifestations of scleroderma, usually in the colon, and they are described as wide-mouthed diverticula on the antimesenteric border formed by mucosa/submucosa bulging through atrophic muscular layer. However pseudosacculation is also described in Crohn's disease as dilated small bowel segment upstream to intestinal strictures.

Suggested Reading

Christensen KN, Fidler JL, Fletcher JG, MacCarty R, Daniel Johnson C (2010) Pictorial review of colonic polyp and mass distortion and recognition with the CT virtual dissection technique. Radiographics 30:5

Elias D, Honoré C, Dumont F, Ducreux M, Boige V, Malka D, Burtin P, Dromain C, Goéré D (2011) Results of systematic second-look surgery plus HIPEC in asymptomatic patients presenting a high risk of developing colorectal peritoneal carcinomatosis. Ann Surg 254(2):289–293

Ho LM, Paulson EK, Thompson WM (2007) Pneumatosis intestinalis in the adult: benign to life-threatening causes. Am J Roentgenol 188:1604–1613

Kim SH, Shin SS, Jeong YY, Heo SH, Kim JW, Kang HK (2009) Gastrointestinal tract perforation: MDCT findings according to the perforation sites. Korean J Radiol 10:63–70

Klaver YL, Lemmens VE, de Hingh IH (2013) Outcome of surgery for colorectal cancer in the presence of peritoneal carcinomatosis. Eur J Surg Oncol 39(7):734–741

Parks AG, Gordon PH, Hardcastle JD (1976) A classification of fistula-in-ano. Br J Surg 63(1):1–12

Reiner CS, Tutuian R, Solopova AE, Pohl D, Marincek B, Weishaupt D (2011) MR defecography in patients with dyssynergic defecation: spectrum of imaging findings and diagnostic value. Br J Radiol 84(998):136–144

Urban BA, Fishman EK (2000) Tailored helical CT evaluation of acute abdomen. Radiographics 20:725–749

Q

No lemma

P. Paolantonio, C. Dromain, *Imaging of Small Bowel, Colon and Rectum*, 129
A-Z Notes in Radiological Practice and Reporting,
DOI 10.1007/978-88-470-5489-9_17, © Springer-Verlag Italia 2014

R

Rectal Carcinoma

- Rectal adenocarcinoma accounts for about 30 % of colorectal cancers. The most common type of rectal cancer is adenocarcinoma, which is a cancer arising from the mucosa. Because of its specific anatomical location, this cancer poses two specific problems in terms of treatment that are the sphincter preservation and locoregional recurrences. The latter depends mainly on the depth of involvement of the rectal wall and mesorectum and of the lymph node involvement.
- Symptoms of rectal carcinoma typically include rectal bleeding and anemia which are sometimes associated with weight loss.
- The indication for treatment is based on the initial assessment of imaging including endorectal ultrasonography, thoracoabdominopelvic CT, and rectal MRI. The aim of imaging is to identify groups of patients with different risk of recurrence

and to choose the most appropriate treatment. It must respond more specifically to three questions:

- What is the exact location of the tumor and the distal margin between the lower pole of the tumor and the sphincter? Its importance is crucial in reaching the lower rectal tumors to assess the possibilities of conservative treatment and thus the potential to preserve continence. Sphincter preservation is possible if you have a distal margin of at least 1 cm.
- What is the stage and the circumferential resection margin? The lateral extension of the tumor is now considered the main risk factor for local recurrence.
- What are the tumor N (nodal) and M (metastases) staging?

• Rigid sigmoidoscopy, corresponding to the insertion of a rigid optical scope inserted through the anus, is usually performed and allows obtaining biopsy specimen and a more exact measurement of the tumor's distance from the anus than flexible sigmoidoscopy. Low, middle, and upper rectal tumors are localized between 0 and 5 cm, 5 and 10 cm, and 10 and 15 cm from the anal margin, respectively. The tumor will be also located in relation to the pouch of Douglas. It is also important to specify the location of the tumor in the axial plane and whether the invasion is circumferential or localized.

• Endorectal ultrasonography is presently the most accurate imaging modality for visualization of the layers of the rectal wall and for the assessment of tumor ingrowth into rectal wall layers with accuracies for T staging varying between 69 and 97 %. However, its sensitivity was shown to be affected by T stage and is higher for staging of superficial rectal tumors (T1 and T2) than for staging of advanced rectal cancer. Moreover, it has a limited value to visualize the mesorectal fascia and to assess the distance from the tumor to this fascia that is, at present, considered to be the most powerful predictor of local recurrence rate.

- MRI has become a complementary tool for the determination of circumferential resection margin particularly useful in the staging of T3 and T4 and to assess the rectal sphincter in tumor of the low rectal cancer. Technically, rectal MRI is based on T2 sequences in the three spatial planes (sagittal, coronal, and oblique axial perpendicular to the long axis of the tumor) without fat saturation to obtain a good contrast between the tumor and the mesorectal fat. Most staging failures with MR imaging occur in the differentiation of T2-stage and borderline T3-stage lesions. Overstaging is often caused by desmoplastic reactions, and it is difficult to distinguish on MR images between spiculation in the perirectal fat caused by fibrosis alone (stage pT2) and spiculation caused by fibrosis that contains tumor cells (stage pT3). Finally for low rectal tumors, it is necessary to evaluate the sphincter complex composed of the levator ani muscle, with a beam ileococcygeal and beam puborectalis, and external and internal sphincters of the anal canal (Fig. 1). This sphincter complex is well depicted using MRI. The levator ani muscle and the external sphincter consist of striated fibers hypointense on T2 sequence, whereas the internal sphincter is a smooth muscle layer following the internal rectal muscularis that strongly enhanced after injection of contrast material.

- Metastatic lymph nodes must be looked for above the level of the tumor. The evaluation of lymph node by imaging is based on morphologic criteria of size and appearance of the lymph nodes. Currently diameters of 5 mm for the mesorectum location and 7 mm for internal iliac location are retained as threshold values for malignant lymph nodes.

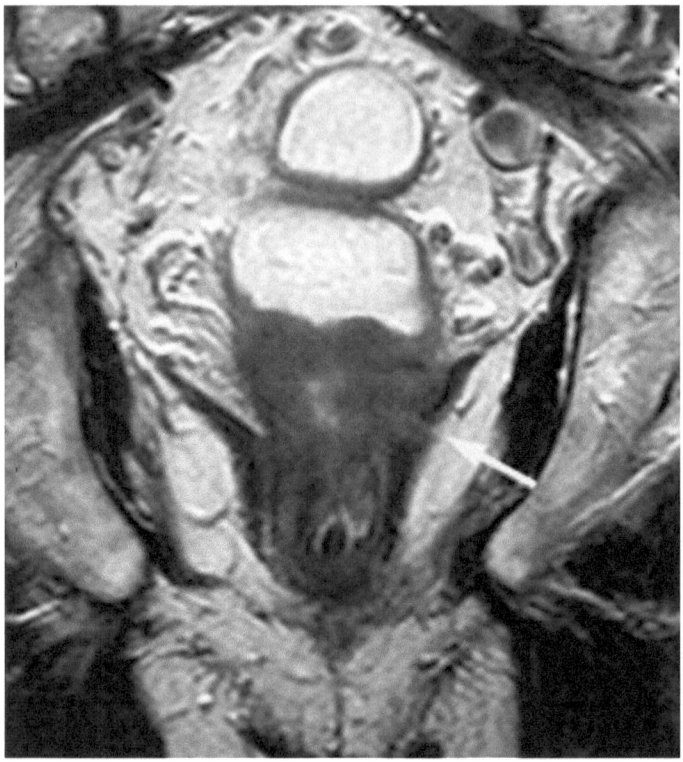

Fig. 1 Rectal adenocarcinoma: Coronal T2-weighted MR image shows a low rectal mass involving the ileococcygeal beam of the levator ani muscle (*arrow*)

- Imaging is also useful to assess response to chemoradiation assessment treatment. MRI is considered as the imaging modality of choice and should be performed 6–8 weeks after the end of treatment. A decrease in T2 signal and volume reduction ≥ 70 % are the signs that are better correlated with histological response and progression-free survival. MR diffusion-weighted sequences improve the performance of MRI to identify tumor remnants and to select the complete response (Fig. 2).

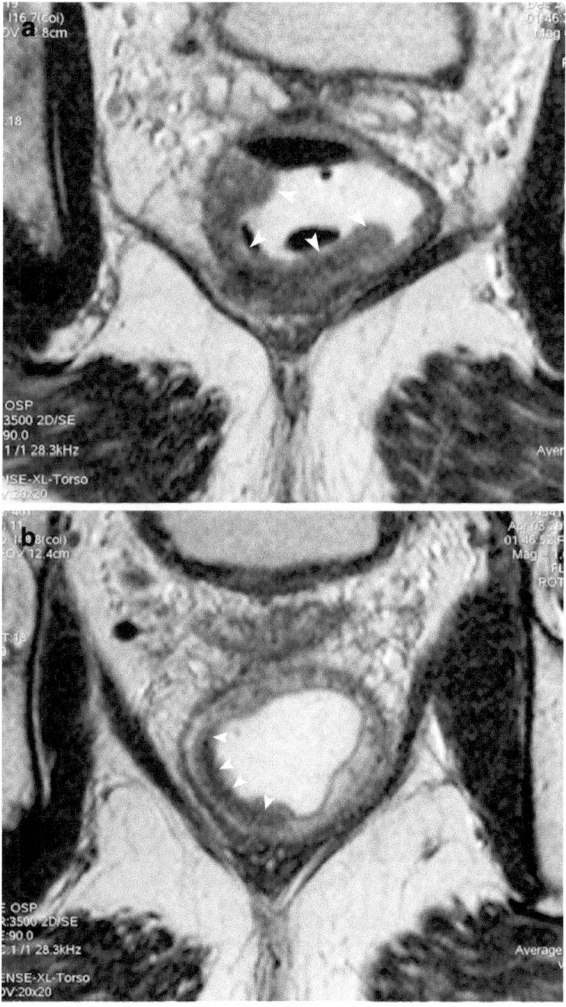

Fig. 2 Rectal adenocarcinoma (*arrowheads*) prior (**a**) and after neoadjuvant chemoradiation (**b**). T2-weighted images depict tumor shrinkage in a patient with complete clinical response. After neoadjuvant chemoradiation, scarring tissue is visible in the tumoral bed (low signal intensity on T2-weighted image and poor signal on heavily diffusion-weighted image) (**c**). (**d**) shows the endoscopic features of mucosal scarring tissue after neoadjuvant therapy

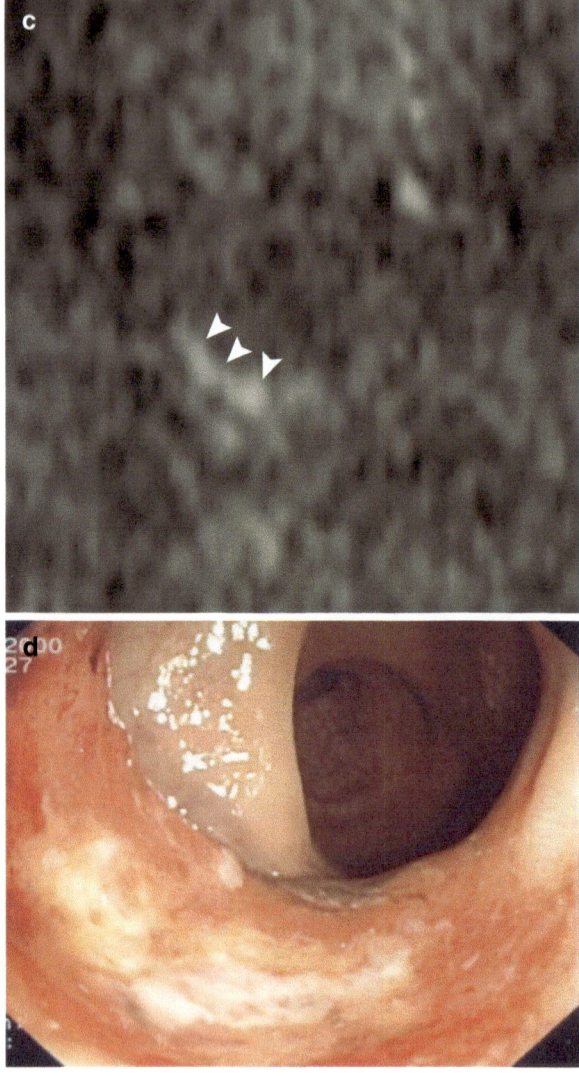

Fig. 2 (continued)

- Neoadjuvant chemoradiotherapy is currently used prior to surgery in rectal carcinoma with mesorectal fascia involvement or with tumor margin close to the mesorectal fascia and mesorectal suspected lymph nodes. Neoadjuvant cht-RTX leads to a complete clinical response in about 30 % of patients.
- The assessment of complete clinical response requires combination of endoscopy and imaging. DW MR imaging in combination with conventional T2-weighted sequence seems to be a promising tool in differentiating between partial response and complete clinical response. In patients with complete clinical response to neoadjuvant therapy, minimal invasive treatment as TEM or wait-and-watch policy have been recently proposed instead of conventional TME; however, these alternative approaches do not reach a complete consensus among the surgical community and are still under clinical investigation.
- The postoperative assessment is based on CT as well as MRI and 18F-FDG PET in cases of difficulties due to fibrotic radiation therapy changes.

Rectal Prolapse

- Rectal prolapse refers to a wide spectrum of conditions characterized by the prolapse of the rectum with respect to its anatomical position associated often with pelvic floor dysfunction. Different types of rectal prolapse can be categorized:
  - *Full-thickness rectal prolapse*
  - *Mucosal rectal prolapse*

depending on the rectal wall layers involved in the prolapse.

Moreover other subclassification is possible considering the degree of prolapse:

- *External prolapse*
- *Internal prolapse*

depending in the rectal wall or the prolapsing mucosa is pulled out of the anus or not during evacuation and straining or at rest.

- Moreover a variant of rectal prolapse is represented by rectal intussusception (either external or internal–occult intussusception). In case of intussusception a proximal prolapsing rectal segment telescopes into a distal rectal segment leading to severe obstruction during defecation. The intussusception can be devised in rectorectal or rectoanal intussusception depending on the segment that hosts the intussuscipiens, the prolapsing rectal segment.

- Rectal prolapse is often associated with rectocele formation and other pelvic organ prolapse (cystocele, colpocele, enterocele) depending on the overall pelvic floor dysfunction.

- Symptoms are represented by various combinations of obstructed defecation, fecal incontinence, hemorrhoids, and rectal ulceration associated sometimes with urinary incontinence.

- Hemorrhoids are quite common in case of rectal prolapse. Recent theory on hemorrhoid pathogenesis postulates that the primum movens of hemorrhoid formation is represented by the presence of redundant and prolapsing rectal mucosa; therefore, one of the modern treatments proposed to care for hemorrhoids as well as rectal prolapse is represented by STARR (stapled transanal rectal resection).

- Imaging plays a role in defining the type and degree of rectal prolapse and the overall pelvic floor dysfunction with relevant impact on patient management considering the different surgical options (STARR, laparoscopic ventral rectopexy, levatorplasty, perineal rectosigmoidectomy with Delmore repair) or possible conservative treatment (dietary prescription and biofeedback training).
- MR defecography represents modern imaging; however, the conventional X-ray defecography still has a role in the accurate assessment of mucosal prolapse.

Rectocele

- Rectocele is defined as bulging or outpouching of the rectal wall during defecation. Usually rectocele involves the anterior rectal wall, and it is common in women (especially after hysterectomy). In anterior rectocele the anterior rectal wall bulges through the rectovaginal septum into the posterior vaginal wall, and it is visible at physical examination. Rectocele is often associated with pelvic floor dysfunction, rectal prolapse, and obstructed defecation syndrome. Rectocele size consists in the measurement of anteroposterior depth of convex wall protrusion extending beyond the expected margin of normal rectal wall: small rectocele (<2 cm), moderate rectocele (2–4 cm), and large rectocele (>4 cm).
- MR defecography represents an accurate radiation-free imaging modality for pelvic floor dysfunction and rectocele measurements (Fig. 3).

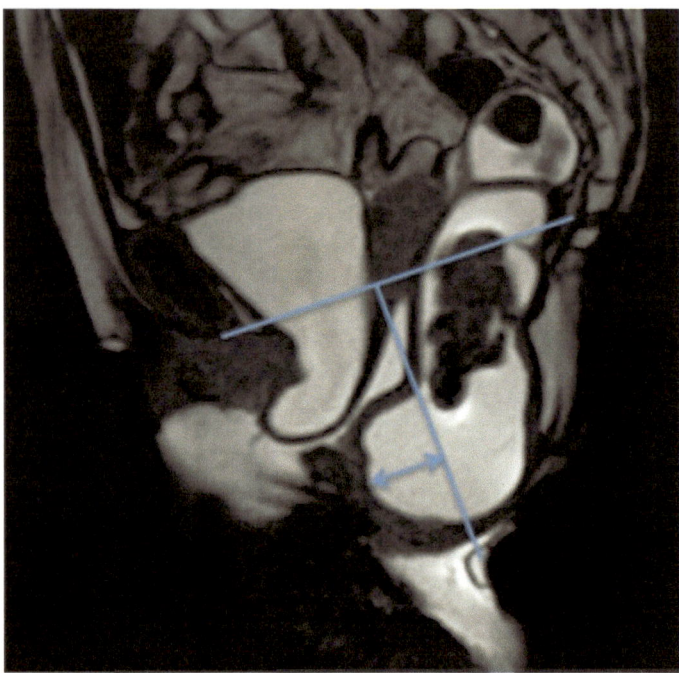

Fig. 3 MR defecography image acquired during defecation phase showing descending perineum with respect to the pubococcygeal line. Anterior rectocele is clearly visible as an anterior bulging of the rectal wall. *Double-arrow line* indicates how to measure rectocele width

Suggested Reading

Beets-Tan RG, Beets GL, Vliegen RF, Kessels AG, Van Boven H, De Bruine A, von Meyenfeldt MF, Baeten CG, van Engelshoven JM (2001) Accuracy of magnetic resonance imaging in prediction of tumour-free resection margin in rectal cancer surgery. Lancet 357(9255):497–504

Brown G, Richards CJ, Bourne MW, Newcombe RG, Radcliffe AG, Dallimore NS, Williams GT (2003) Morphologic predictors of lymph node statue in rectal cancer with use of High-spatial-resolution MR Imaging with histopathologic comparison. Radiology 227(2):371–377

Iafrate F, Laghi A, Paolantonio P, Rengo M, Mercantini P, Ferri M, Ziparo V, Passariello R (2006) Preoperative staging of rectal cancer with MR Imaging: correlation with surgical and histopathologic findings. Radiographics 26(3):701–714

MERCURY Study Group (2007) Extramural depth of tumor invasion at thin-section MR in patients with rectal cancer: results of the MERCURY study. Radiology 243(1):132–139

Ptok H, Ruppert R, Stassburg J, Maurer CA, Oberholzer K, Junginger T, Merkel S, Hermanek P (2013) Pretherapeutic MRI for decision-making regarding selective neoadjuvant radiochemotherapy for rectal carcinoma: interim analysis of a multicentric prospective observational study. J Magn Reson Imaging 37(5):1122–1128

Seynaeve P, Billiet I, Vossaert P, Verleyen P, Steegmans A (2006) MR imaging of the pelvic floor. JBR 89:182–189

S

Sandwich Sign

- The sandwich sign refers to the cross-sectional imaging appearance, most often on CT examination, of mesenteric fat and vessels as the sandwich filling, while the homogeneous soft tissue adenopathy represents sandwich bun.
- The sandwich sign is due to the presence of large bulky mesenteric adenopathy and is specific to mesenteric lymphomas. Mesenteric lymphomas are unique because they can grow to a large size and can envelop fat, bowel, and vessels without causing clinical symptoms. Most of these mesenteric lymphomas are NHLs. However in patients who have undergone transplantation, PTLD (posttransplant lymphoproliferative disorder), an Epstein–Barr virus-driven B-cell lymphoproliferation in immunosuppressed patients who have undergone transplantation can also create a sandwich sign.

P. Paolantonio, C. Dromain, *Imaging of Small Bowel, Colon and Rectum*, 143
A-Z Notes in Radiological Practice and Reporting,
DOI 10.1007/978-88-470-5489-9_19, © Springer-Verlag Italia 2014

Scleroderma, GI Tract

- Scleroderma is a disease of unknown etiology characterized by widespread disorder of microvasculature and overproduction of collagen causing exuberant interstitial fibrosis with atrophy and sclerosis of many organs and systems; the skin is the most common affected tissue.
- However important gastrointestinal manifestations of scleroderma are described: esophageal manifestation is quite common (hypotonia and aperistalsis and dysphagia), followed by stomach involvement (gastric dilatation, delayed empty), small bowel (malabsorption due to bacterial overgrowth and delayed transit time and jejunal dilatation with pseudosacculation due to smooth muscle atrophy) and colon (constipation with pseudosacculation, complete loss of haustration, and marked dilatation, bacterial overgrowth, and cystic pneumatosis).
- In case of small bowel involvement, the duodenal and jejunal dilatation may simulate a small bowel obstruction leading to a misdiagnosis and unnecessary exploratory surgery.

Sigmoid Volvulus

- Sigmoid volvulus usually affects elderly patients presenting with anatomical long sigmoid mesentery (Fig. 1). Sigmoid twist on mesenteric axis, the degree of torsion is variable (from 180° to 360° up to 540°). Twisted sigmoid colon appears as a greatly distended paralyzed loop (coffee bean sign at plain X-ray), with inverted U-shaped distended sigmoid colon and absence of air in the rectum detectable at CT scout view.

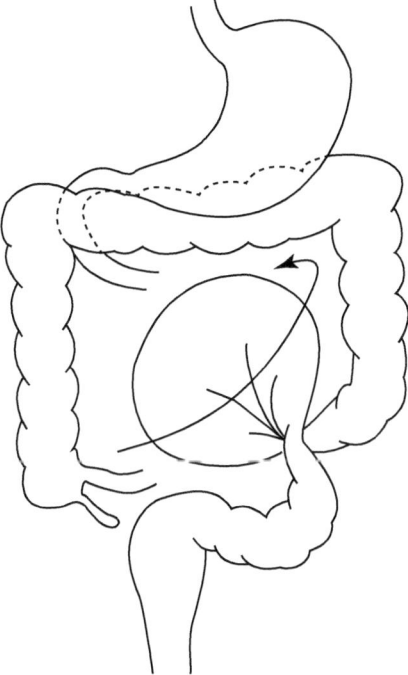

Fig. 1 Graphic illustrates the mechanism of sigmoid volvulus formation due to torsion and various degrees of rotation of the sigmoid colon with respect to the sigmoid mesentery

- At CT the presence of distended sigmoid colon with two transition zones in the same point is the sign of a severe sigmoid twisting. Whirl sign with tightly torsioned mesentery formed by twisted afferent plus efferent loop is another sign of severe twisting.

Situs Viscerum Inversus

- Situs viscerum inversus is a congenital malposition (complete or partial) of organs. It can be associated or not with Kartagener syndrome (autosomal recessive disease with defective cilia motility leading to situs viscerum inversus, chronic sinusitis, and bronchiectasia). Considering the bowel the malposition of the gastrointestinal tract is referred as partial or complete intestinal malrotation. Important anatomical landmark in case of intestinal malrotation is represented by positioning of the third portion of duodenum and Treitz ligament, positioning of jejunal loop, and the site of the cecum.

Small Bowel Benign Tumor

- Benign tumor are quite rare in the small bowel. Leiomyoma is the most common benign tumor of small bowel. This is a benign smooth muscle tumor that arises in approximately 50 % of cases in the jejunum, followed by the ileum. Almost one half of all lesions are less than 5 cm. Other types of benign small bowel tumor are lipomas, angiomas, adenomas, neurofibromas, and fibromas.
- In 50 % of cases the tumor is asymptomatic. Otherwise, the common clinical presentation is a history of bleeding from the bowel, anemia, and obstruction. Bleeding is less frequent in case of lipomas which are predominantly developed in the ileum with a high incidence of intussusceptions.
- CT enteroclysis which combines the advantages of CT (extraluminal information) and conventional enteroclysis (distension of small bowel and lumen content analysis) is the imaging modality of choice for the detection of small bowel tumors. However it has a variable value. Indeed, intramural lesions that were totally in the wall of the bowel could be missed. Submucosal tumor

produces filling defect, whereas subserosal tumor grows larger and has most often an exophytic component. Leiomyomas have a median size of 5 cm at time of diagnosis, round shape, sharp margins, and homogeneous density. Calcifications are occasionally detected. Intestinal lipomas are well-circumscribed masses of fat tissue with low CT density arising within the submucosa and occasionally surrounded by a capsule.

- Video capsule endoscopy (VCE) and double-balloon endoscopy (DBE) have recently been introduced in clinical practice, to evaluate obscure bleeding in the small intestine. VCE is intended mainly to screen patients because it is not invasive. On the other hand, DBE is often the first diagnostic modality when a small bowel lesion is strongly suggested. Moreover DBE allows to perform biopsies and to determine the most appropriate surgical approach.

Small Bowel Malignant Tumor

- Malignant neoplasms of the small bowel are among the rarest types of cancer, accounting for only 2 % of all GI cancers. Adenocarcinoma, lymphoma (see lymphoma), and carcinoid tumors (see carcinoid) account for the majority of small intestine malignancies. Adenocarcinoma is the most common histological type. Its prevalence tends to increase with age, with a mean age at diagnosis of approximately 60 years. Similar to adenocarcinomas in the colon, those in the small bowel arise from premalignant adenomas occurring both sporadically and in the context of familial adenomatous polyposis. Approximately 50 % arise in the duodenum, 30 % in the jejunum, and 20 % in the ileum. Leiomyosarcoma is an extremely rare malignant mesenchymal tumor of smooth muscle and accounts for between 5 and 10 % of soft tissue sarcomas. They should be differentiated from gastrointestinal stromal tumors (GISTs) that are often CD34 immunoreactive and express tyrosine kinase c-kit (CD117) receptor activity, in contrast to leiomyosarcomas.

- Small bowel cancer is typically asymptomatic in its early stages. Nausea, vomiting, and intestinal obstruction are common presenting symptoms but unfortunately reflect advanced disease.
- Upper GI endoscopy with small bowel enteroscopy (push enteroscopy) may identify and allow biopsy of lesions in the duodenum and jejunum. Colonoscopy with retrograde ileoscopy may be useful in identifying ileal tumors.
- Standard abdominal CT scan had a limited sensitivity to detect the tumor. To increase its sensitivity, CT enteroclysis which combines the advantages of CT (extraluminal information) and conventional enteroclysis (distension of small bowel) is the imaging method of choice for the diagnostic and local staging. Adenocarcinomas have a weak enhancement, opposite to endocrine and stromal tumors, and are often stenosing. Leiomyosarcomas are larger (average, 12 cm) than the leiomyomas and have an irregular shape, predominantly exophytic, and have a nonhomogeneous appearance both before and after contrast enhancement (Fig. 2). Some lesions have central zones of liquefaction. The tumor heterogeneity seems to be the most specific in suggesting a malignant neoplasm.
- CT is also essential for the pretreatment staging and follow-up of these lesions. More common metastatic sites are the liver, abdominal lymphadenopathy, peritoneum, and lung.
- Video capsule endoscopy (VCE) and double-balloon endoscopy (DBE) have recently been introduced in clinical practice, to assist in the evaluation of small bowel tumors, and are recommended in case of bleeding of unknown origin, which persists or recurs after negative findings of initial or primary endoscopy, namely, colonoscopy and/or upper endoscopy. DBE allows to perform biopsies and to determine the most appropriate surgical approach.

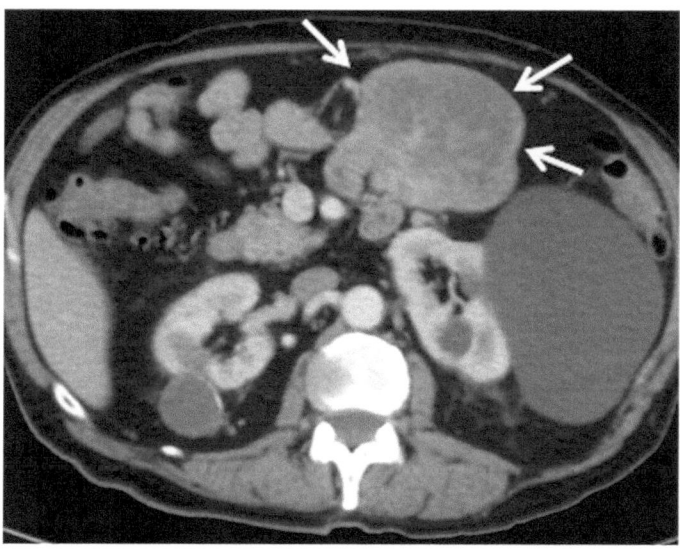

Fig. 2 Leiomyosarcoma of the small bowel. Axial contrast-enhanced CT images show a large and heterogeneous exophytic mass developing from the small bowel (*arrows*)

Small Bowel Metastases

- Small bowel metastases are extremely rare and represent less than 10 % of malignant tumors of the small bowel. The most frequent sites of primary lesions are the uterus, uterine cervix, and colon, which are the adjacent organs to the small intestine. Other common sites resulting from hematogenous dissemination of the disease and contributing to intestinal metastasis are the lung, breast, kidney, bladder, and ovary, and melanoma skin cancers.
- Although intestinal metastases are a frequent autopsy finding, they rarely become clinically apparent. The signs and symptoms largely depend on the site of the metastatic tumor.

- Metastatic disease to the small intestine may present with acute or subacute intestinal obstruction, ileus, gastrointestinal hemorrhage, or bowel perforation which may be complicated by peritonitis. Sometimes it is an incidental finding depicted during FDG PET-CT follow-up. It is seen that jejunal metastasis is rather complicated by perforation, while ileal metastatic lesions are more obstructive.
- Upper gastrointestinal endoscopy can be used to diagnose proximal lesions. More distal lesion can be depicted using CT enteroclysis with 97 % sensitivity and 80 % of specificity in detecting primary and secondary small bowel tumor.
- Similar to primary small intestine tumors, small bowel metastases can have various radiologic appearances including thickening of the bowel wall, mass effect, and nodular filling defects. Excavation of a small intestinal metastatic mass has also been reported. Lesions are often multiples. Role of FDG PET-CT and capsule endoscopy in diagnosing metastatic small bowel disease is still being explored with some early success (Fig. 3).

Small Bowel Diverticula

- Small bowel diverticula can be categorized as true diverticula (duodenal diverticula, jejunal diverticulosis, and Meckel diverticulum) and pseudodiverticula (scleroderma, Crohn's disease, lymphoma, mesenteric ischemia, communicating ileal duplication).

Small Bowel Duplication Cyst

- Small bowel duplication cyst is the most common duplication cyst of the alimentary tract, and it becomes symptomatic usually

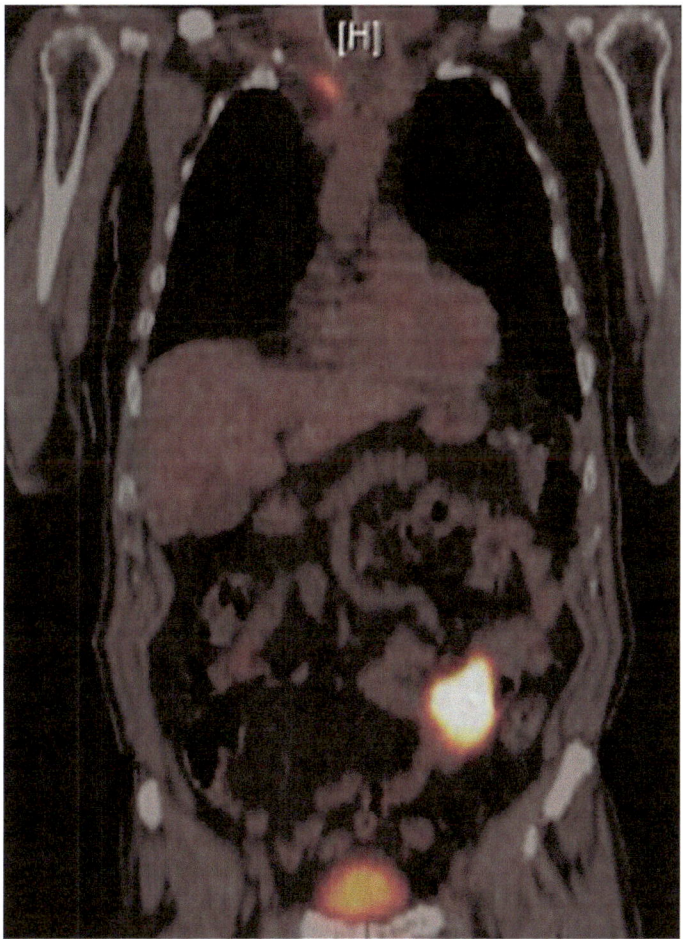

Fig. 3 Small bowel metastasis from a thyroid cancer. Coronal FDG PET image shows an intense tracer uptake fixation in a small bowel loop

in the neonatal period. Cyst contains gastric ectopic mucosa or ectopic pancreatic tissue. Small bowel duplication cyst may develop in small bowel obstruction due to intussusceptions.

Small Bowel Wall Thickening

- Cross-sectional imaging (either CT or MRI) enables to assess the small bowel wall thickness and to measure it. Normal bowel wall thickness depends by the degree of luminal distension.
- When a good luminal distension is achieved (CT/MR enterography/enteroclysis or conventional CT/MR scan with intrinsic bowel lumen distension), the normal bowel wall is very thin (1–2 mm). However in case of nondistended or collapsed intestinal loop, a bowel wall thickness of 3 mm should be considered as normal.
- Bowel wall thickening is a very aspecific finding since it may be related to a number of entities including normal variants, inflammatory conditions, and neoplastic disease.
  Therefore in case of bowel wall thickening, other findings should be accurately analyzed such as *pattern of attenuation* (intramural high density or air density or fat density) and *contrast-enhancement pattern* (homogeneous, low or lacking bowel wall enhancement, hyper-enhancement, target appearance), *degree of thickening* (mild, moderate, marked), *pattern of thickening* (symmetric vs. asymmetric thickening, focal vs. diffuse, segmental distribution), associated *perienteric abnormalities* (fat stranding, lymph nodes, mesenteric vessel engorgement, abscesses, fistulas, peritoneal fluids). A comprehensive evaluation of all these parameters and an accurate comparison with clinical and laboratoristic data will lead to a more accurate differential diagnosis. Same considerations are also valid for large bowel wall thickening.
- In general diffuse symmetric bowel wall thickening with target appearance after contrast medium injection associated with perienteric findings (marked fat stranding) suggests an inflammatory origin, while focal asymmetric thickening with poor perivisceral modification suggests a neoplastic origin.

Some findings may suggest a definite diagnosis of Crohn's disease (segmentary bowel involvement with thickening of mesenteric fat, comb sign, cobblestoning, target enhancement). Some findings such as colonic accordion sign suggest an acute inflammatory colitis. Fat deposit into the bowel wall suggests a chronic inflammation of the bowel

- Pneumatosis according to clinical data suggests the bowel wall infarction.
- A marked focal wall thickening with homogeneous appearance of bowel wall, poor perivisceral modification, and bowel lumen pseudodilatation may suggest the diagnosis of bowel lymphoma.

String Sign

- String sign is the sign of a small bowel stricture in Crohn's disease patients due to marked narrowing of rigid loops.

STARR

- Stapled transanal rectal resection is a minimally invasive surgical procedure performed using transanal dedicated circular stapler instruments allowing resection of redundant rectal tissue responsible of rectal prolapse, hemorrhoid formation, and obstructed defecation syndrome without external incision with prompt patient recovery and less postoperative pain with respect to conventional hemorrhoidectomy. This technique was firstly described by Longo, an Italian surgeon, and has been widely adopted for treating prolapsed hemorrhoids instead of conventional hemorrhoidectomy as well as to treat obstructed defecation syndrome caused by rectocele, rectal prolapse, and rectal invagination. STARR is contraindicated in patients with anismus, pelvic floor incoordination, and enterocele due to the higher rate of complications. Therefore accurate imaging of the pelvic floor is suggested in selecting patients for STARR using MR defecography or conventional X-ray defecography.

Suggested Reading

Bhavsar AS, Verma S, Lamba R, Lall CG, Koenigsknecht V, Rajesh A (2013) Abdominal manifestations of neurologic disorders. Radiographics 33(1):135–153

Corman ML, Carriero A, Hager T, Herold A, Jayne DG, Lehur P-A, Lomanto D, Longo A, Mellgren AF, Nicholls J, Nyström P-O, Senagore AJ, Stuto A, Wexner SD (2006) Consensus conference on the stapled transanal rectal resection (STARR) for disordered defaecation. Colorectal Dis 8(2):98–101

Hardy SM (2003) The sandwich sign. Radiology 226(3):651–652

Levsky JM, Den EI, DuBrow RA, Wolf EL, Rozenblit AM (2010) CT findings of sigmoid volvulus. AJR 194:136–143

Macari M, Balthazar EJ (2001) CT of bowel wall thickening: significance and pitfalls of interpretation. AJR 176:1105–1116

Masselli G, Casciani E, Polettini E, Laghi F, Gualdi G (2013) Magnetic resonance imaging of small bowel neoplasms. Cancer Imaging 13:92–99

Medappil N, Reghukumar R (2010) Sandwich sign in mesenteric lymphoma. J Cancer Res Ther 6(3):403–404

Megibow AJ, Balthazar EJ, Hulnick DH, Naidich DP, Bosniak MA (1985) CY evaluation of gastrointestinal leiomyomas and leiomyosarcoma. AJR 144(4):727–731

Pilleul F, Penigaud M, Milot L, Saurin JC, Chayvialle JA, Valette PJ (2006) Possible small-bowel neoplasm: contrast-enhanced and water-enhanced multidetector CT enteroclysis. Radiology 241(3):796–801

Taenia

- Taenia also called tapeworm is a parasite (cyclophillidean cestode); it infects pigs and humans and pigs are intermediate host.
- Taenia infection is caused by ingestion of eggs shed in the feces of a human tapeworm carrier. Adult tapeworms develop (up to 2–7 m in length and produce less than 1,000 proglottids, each with approximately 50,000 eggs) and reside in the small intestine for years. Small bowel exams (X-ray follow-through and MR enterography) are able to detect a filling defect into the small bowel lumen. However diagnosis is made possible detecting proglottids or eggs in the stool.

Tailgut Cyst

- Tailgut cyst or retrorectal cystic hamartoma is a congenital cyst due to incomplete regression of embryonic tailgut (distal portion of the gut). It appears in imaging as a thin-walled multicystic or unilocular cyst in the presacral space adhering

P. Paolantonio, C. Dromain, *Imaging of Small Bowel, Colon and Rectum*,   155
A-Z Notes in Radiological Practice and Reporting,
DOI 10.1007/978-88-470-5489-9_20, © Springer-Verlag Italia 2014

to sacrum, rectum, or both with extension into the ischiorectal fossa.

- Tailgut cyst may be asymptomatic or lead to rectal pain, rectal bleeding, or urinary frequency. Average age at diagnosis is 35 years, and it is more commonly reported in females.
- Differential diagnosis should consider perirectal abscess with anorectal fistula and mucinous adenocarcinoma and can be performed on cytological or histological basis. At drainage mucoid fluid is present and not pus.
- MRI is the imaging modality of choice using phased-array coil, TSE T2-weighted sequences and contrast-enhanced T1-weighted fat saturation allowing accurate anatomical details and assessment of cyst wall in order to rule out enhancing mural nodularity/septa that may suggest the diagnosis of mucinous adenocarcinoma.
- At histology tailgut cyst shows several types of epithelia plus smooth muscle.

Target Sign

- Target sign is referred as a stratified appearance, a bowel segment, or a stratified enhancement pattern of bowel wall detectable at cross-sectional imaging when image is acquired orthogonal to bowel loop so that its thickened bowel wall appears as multiple concentric rings with different attenuation/signal intensity or different degrees of contrast enhancement.
- Target sign was firstly described by Balthazar in 1991 using CT imaging referring to a contrast-enhancement pattern of a symmetric thickened bowel wall presenting three layers (inner enhancing layer, outer enhancing layer, intermediate layer with reduced attenuation with respect to the enhancing

layers). The explanation of these findings regards different degrees of inflammation and edema of the bowel wall with hyperemia of the mucosa (inner enhancing layer) and serosa/muscularis propria (outer layer) with edema of submucosa (intermediate non-enhancing layer). The target sign is best appreciable on arterial and portal venous phase; in case of marked submucosa edema, it can be detected also at non-enhanced study. The same enhancement pattern is detectable also at MRI with the same meaning. Inner low attenuation layer may also represent fatty deposit into submucosa layer (check quantitatively HU at non-enhanced CT or analyze SI on T1-weighted and fat-suppressed T1-weighted MR images) and is associated to chronic inflammation (proctitis after radiation therapy or ulcerative colitis or Crohn's disease).

- While nonspecific the target sign may allow to suggest the inflammatory origin of bowel wall thickening.
- Target sign is described in several conditions, most of them addressed as inflammatory changes of bowel wall (appendicitis, CMV colitis, Crohn's disease, Henoch–Schonlein purpura, ischemic enteritis or colitis, pseudomembranous colitis, radiation-induced enteritis, ulcerative colitis, and bowel edema associated with portal hypertension). However also intussusception showed a target appearance due to the concentric "telescopic" configuration of intussuscipiens and intussusceptum bowel wall and mesenteric fat.

TEM

- Transanal endoscopic microsurgery (TEM) is a minimally invasive surgical technique, which is performed endoluminally and is optically enhanced (usually through stereoscopic vision). This is an organ preservation technique with local excision (disc excision) of the rectal wall without lymph node removal that allows the patient to recover rapidly. The whole procedure is performed transanally.

- It is primarily used for the removal of benign rectal tumors particularly for elderly and unfit patients. This treatment has been also proposed for the treatment of T1 low-risk rectal cancer with local recurrence rates of approximately 5 %. An extension of the indication is controversially discussed in T2 and T3 rectal tumors in combination with radiochemotherapy.
- Accurate staging using endorectal ultrasound and MRI is essential for the selection of patients. TEM is an alternative treatment of the resection of rectal lesions to more radical surgery associated with minimal morbidity and mortality and improved functional outcome. However this technique does not allow a definite operative staging and is associated with higher local recurrence rates.

Total Mesorectal Excision

- The total mesorectal excision is a surgical treatment of reference for rectal cancer. It was introduced in 1982 by the surgeon Richard John Heald. It consists in a total mesorectal excision which involves complete removal of the tumor along with the mesorectal tissue. In TME the entire mesorectal compartment including the rectum, surrounding mesorectal fat, perirectal lymph nodes, and its envelope, i.e., the mesorectal fascia, is completely removed. This minimizes the chance of tumor remnants in the surgical bed. It is considered as a major advancement in the treatment of rectal cancer and is associated with a drop in local recurrence rates from 40 to 11 %.

Trauma, GI Tract

- Gastrointestinal tract is involved in blunt trauma in 5 % of cases, more frequently in children (lap belts, bicycle handlebar injuries, or child abuse).
- Location of intestinal traumatic lesion is in the proximal jejunum followed in frequency by the duodenum, ascending colon at the ileocecal valve, and descending colon.
- At non-enhanced CT pneumoperitoneum is easily detected (small gas bubble anteriorly near the liver/trapped within leaves of mesentery) (see also perforation). Retroperitoneal air suggests the perforation of the duodenum or colon. Free fluid is commonly seen. A "sentinel" high-density clot adjacent to bowel loops may also seen.
- At contrast-enhanced CT, a focal discontinuity of bowel wall representing the direct evidence of bowel wall disruption should be accurately researched. Moreover, a focal wall thickening (>3 mm) may be a sign of intramural hematoma. Injured bowel wall may also show an increased contrast enhancement due to delayed venous transit time.
- Mesenteric abnormalities after trauma can be easily detected at CT (mesenteric hematoma or mesenteric fat stranding with streaky hyperattenuation due to hemorrhage, infiltration, and inflammation).

Tuberculosis, GI Tract

- Intestinal tuberculosis is rarely encountered in western countries and is commonly associated with pulmonary manifestations in immunocompromised patients.
- Location of intestinal tuberculosis is represented by ileocecal area, ascending colon, jejunum, appendix, duodenum, stomach, sigmoid, and rectum in descending frequency.

- From a pathology point of view, two forms of intestinal TBC are categorized: ulcerative form and hypertrophic form.
- Tubercular peritonitis may result from rupture of mesenteric node, or hematogenous spread may evolve in generalized abdominal abscesses.
  Several types of tubercular peritonitis are described:

  – Wet type: exudative ascites with high protein and leukocyte contents (large amount of free fluid or loculated fluid collection)
  – High-density ascites (20–45 HU) due to high protein and cellular content
  – Dry or plastic type: caseous adenopathy and adhesion
  – Fibrotic–fixed type: omental cake mass and loops fixation

- At CT the ileocecal area is the most common localization of TBC (due to abundance of lymphoid tissue) showing a circumferential wall thickening of cecum and terminal ileum wall or an asymmetric thickening of ileocecal valve and medial cecal wall with engulfing terminal ileum.
- Differential diagnosis should consider other causes of terminal ileum and cecal wall thickening such as Crohn's disease, amebiasis, and cecal carcinoma.
- However an important finding suggesting the tubercular ileitis is represented by the presence of enlarged mesenteric lymph node with central hypodense area (caseous necrosis).

Typhlitis

- Typhlitis (neutropenic colitis) is an acute inflammation of the cecum, appendix, and occasionally terminal ileum described in patients with leukemia and severe neutropenia.

The terms originate from the Greek word "typhlos" that means blind sac (cecum).

- It represents an acute inflammatory disease of the cecum caused by infectious disease (CMV, candida, *Klebsiella*, *E. coli*, *B. fragilis*, *Enterobacter*), leukemic/lymphomatous infiltrate, ischemia, or focal pseudomembranous colitis.

Suggested Reading

Ahualli J (2005) The target sign: Bowel wall. Radiology 234:549–550

Bokkerink GMJ, de Graaf EJR, de Punt CJ et al (2011) The CARTS study: chemoradiation therapy for rectal cancer in the distal rectum followed by organ-sparing transanal endoscopic microsurgery. BMC Surg 11:34

Iafrate F, Laghi A, Paolantonio P, Rengo M, Mercantini P, Ferri M, Ziparo V, Passariello R (2006) Preoperative staging of rectal cancer with MR Imaging: correlation with surgical and histopathologic findings. Radiographics 26(3):701–714

Joseph DK, Kunac A, Kinler RL, Staff I, Butler KL (2013) Diagnosing blunt hollow viscus injury: is computed tomography the answer? Am J Surg 205(4):414–418

Kunitake H, Abbas MA (2012) Transanal endoscopic microsurgery for rectal tumors: a review. Perm J 16(2):45–50

Paolantonio P, Rengo M, Iafrate F, Martino G, Laghi A (2006) Diagnosis of Taenia saginata by MR enterography. AJR 187:238–243

Suri S, Gupta S, Suri R (1999) Computed tomography in abdominal tuberculosis. Br J Radiol 72:92–98

Vogel MN, Goeppert B, Maksimovic O, Brodoefel H, Faul C, Claussen CD, Horger M (2010) CT features of neutropenic enterocolitis in adult patients with hematological diseases undergoing chemotherapy. Rofo 182(12):1076–1081

Yang DM, Park CH, Jin W, Chang SK, Kim JE, Choi SJ, Jung DH (2005) Tailgut cyst: MRI evaluation. AJR 184:1519–1523

U

Ulcerative Colitis

- Ulcerative colitis is a common chronic idiopathic inflammatory bowel disease with continuous concentric symmetric colonic involvement (prevalence 50–80/100.000).
- At pathology a dominant involvement of mucosa and submucosa is reported with edema and cryptic abscess resulting in shallow ulceration.
- Alternating periods of remission and exacerbation of bloody diarrhea, fever, and abdominal cramps represent clinical findings. Extracolic manifestations are iritis, erythema nodosum, primary sclerosing cholangitis, and spondylitis.
- Ulcerative colitis begins in the rectum with proximal progression.
- In some patients the inflammatory process involves the entire colon (pancolitis).
- Terminal ileum is often inflamed due to reflux of fecal material from the cecum to the ileum (backwash ileitis).

- Patients affected by ulcerative colitis show an increased risk to develop colon adenocarcinoma (risk starts after 8–10 years from the disease's onset, and it is higher in patients with pancolitis).
- Optical colonoscopy and biopsy play a crucial role in diagnosis, follow-up, and surveillance for colon cancer early diagnosis.
- At barium enema, several findings are described in different stage disease:
    - Acute phase: lumen narrowing (spasm), fine mucosal irregularities, hazy bowel contour, ulcers, and "thumbprinting" (symmetric thickening of colonic folds and pseudopolyps and presacral space widening).
    - Subacute phase: haustra distortion, inflammatory polyps, and granular mucosa
    - Chronic stage: loss of haustration, shortening of the colon, "burn-out" colon (fairly distensible colon without haustra), post-inflammatory polyps (filiform polyps), and backwash ileitis.

- Optical colonoscopy completely replaced X-ray conventional studies in diagnosis and follow-up of ulcerative colitis owing to a better assessment of mucosal abnormalities and the advantage to perform a biopsy with histological analysis of colonic mucosa.
- At CT imaging the unique nonspecific findings of ulcerative colitis is represented by large bowel wall thickening (<10 mm).
  Imaging still plays an important role in ulcerative colitis complication such as toxic megacolon (see toxic megacolon) and perforation.
- In early stage of disease, especially in young adults and children, a definite differential diagnosis with Crohn's disease (Crohn's colitis) may be not easy based on clinical, endoscopic, and histological findings owing to a certain degree of

finding overlap. In children a third form of chronic inflammatory bowel disease was categorized, the so-called indeterminate-type colitis, when a clear differential diagnosis is not reached. In this setting imaging (MR/CT enteroclysis/enterography) as well as capsule endoscopy is used to investigate accurately the small bowel since the presence of affected small bowel (with the exception of backwash ileitis) suggests a Crohn's disease diagnosis. Other findings suggesting Crohn's disease are related to the segmental and eccentricity of mucosal and bowel wall involvement and presence of deep ulcers and fistulas.

Ulcerative Jejunoileitis

- Ulcerative jejunoileitis is an acute complicating lesion of refractory celiac disease.

Suggested Reading

De Tomas J, Munoz Caiero A, Gonzalex LV (1994) Ulcerative jejunitis: a complication of celiac disease. Rev ESP Enferm Dig 86(4):761–763
Kirsner JB (1991) Inflammatory bowel disease. Part II: clinical and therapeutic aspects. Dis Mon 37(11):669–746

V

Vasculitis, GI Tract

- Vasculitis can cause local or diffuse pathological changes in the gastrointestinal tract, resulting in nonspecific paralytic ileus, mesenteric ischemia, submucosal edema and hemorrhage, or bowel perforation or stricture.
- The extent and clinical course of disease depend on the size and location of the affected vessel and the histological characteristics of the lesion. Vasculitis may primarily involve large vessels (e.g., giant cell arteritis, Takayasu arteritis), medium-sized vessels (e.g., polyarteritis nodosa, Kawasaki disease, primary granulomatous central nervous system vasculitis), or small vessels (e.g., Wegener granulomatosis, Churg–Strauss syndrome, microscopic polyangiitis, Henoch–Schönlein syndrome, systemic lupus erythematosus, rheumatoid vasculitis, Behçet syndrome). Most of them may show gastrointestinal involvement.
- Radiologic findings in various types of vasculitis often overlap considerably and therefore have limited value in making a specific diagnosis. Nevertheless, the possibility of vasculitis should be considered whenever mesenteric ischemic changes

occur in young patients, are noted at unusual sites (e.g., stomach, duodenum, rectum), and have a tendency to concomitantly involve the small and large intestine and when differential diagnosis with more common disease presenting with similar findings is ruled out.

Therefore clinical findings and lab test as well as biopsy and histology on target organ are crucial to reach the correct diagnosis.

- In *polyarteritis nodosa* the kidneys are the most common involved organs: however, gastrointestinal tract and more commonly the small bowel is the second target of this necrotizing vasculitis. Imaging findings overlap with those of acute mesenteric ischemia, and multiple mesenteric renal, hepatic, and splenic pseudoaneurysm can be detected using CT angiography or more easily with conventional angiography.

- In *Wegener granulomatosis* the target organs are represented by the lung and airways, although intestinal manifestation mimics inflammatory bowel disease.

- In *Churg–Strauss syndrome*, the lung is commonly involved by a granulomatous vasculitis that typically shows three phases: allergic rhinitis and asthma, peripheral eosinophilia (with eosinophilic pneumonia and gastroenteritis), and systemic small vessel granulomatous vasculitis.

- In *microscopic polyangiitis* findings are very similar to polyarteritis nodosa with smaller vessel involvement.

- *Henoch-Schönlein syndrome* is a hypersensitivity-related small vessel acute vasculitis more common in children and young adults with frequent gastrointestinal and cutaneous manifestation (purpuric rush) associated with arthralgia and hematuria.

- *Systemic lupus erythematosus* is an autoimmune disease affecting the musculoskeletal system, kidney, skin, and gastrointestinal tract; diagnosis is performed using well-defined clinical criteria. GI manifestation is common and may involve each section of the GI tract with gastrointestinal ischemia, ulceration, infarction, and perforation.

- *Behçet syndrome* is a nonspecific necrotizing vasculitis with well-defined multiorgan involvement including orogenital ulcers, uveitis, arthritis, neurologic, and gastrointestinal disorders. The hallmark of Behçet syndrome in the gastrointestinal tract is the presence of deep penetrating ulceration of mucosa, submucosa, and even muscular layer as results an high percentage of perforation, hemorrhage, fistulas, and peritonitis have been reported. At CT the intestinal segment involved shows concentric bowel wall thickening or polypoid mass with marked contrast enhancement.

Villous Adenoma, Colon

- Villous adenoma of the colon is a rare benign tumor accounting from 0.1 to 7 % of all rectal and sigmoid lesions. Although this is a benign lesion, it has a strong tendency toward invasion and malignant transformation in 15–25 %. The term "villous tumor" was originated by Holmes in 1860 and has been previously called papillomas, mucous or columnar papillomas, villous papillomas, papillary polyps or adenomas, villous adenomas, and villomas. These adenomas occur more frequently in the rectum and rectosigmoid, although they may occur anywhere in the colon. Although rare, villous adenomas of the duodenum and the small bowel, particularly at the ampulla, can occur. However, similar lesions have been described in the stomach and gallbladder.
- Although the adenomatous polyp is typically a compact, spheroid, pedunculated mass, the villous adenoma is a soft, sessile tumor without a pedicle. It ranges in size from a nodule several centimeters in diameter to a mass of enormous size, completely encircling the bowel.

- The most prominent and characteristic symptom is the profuse discharge of large amounts of mucus produced by the tumor. Occasionally, in case or rectal location, a palpable mass is present upon digital rectal examination.
- On fecal blood testing (hemoccult) only 20–40 % of patients with adenomas have positive test findings, usually resulting from distal and larger polyps.
- Endoscopy is the most sensitive method and the first-line procedure of choice of diagnosing villous polyps. Moreover, it also allows therapeutic intervention. The sensitivity for detecting polyps by colonoscopy is 94 %. Villous adenomas at colonoscopy are usually bulky, sessile, soft, velvety, and friable. Enteroscopy is used to help investigate for small bowel adenomas.

VIPoma

- VIPoma is a pancreatic neuroendocrine tumor which secretes vasoactive intestinal peptide (VIP). These tumors arise in the pancreas 90 % of the time but have also been described in the colon, bronchus, and adrenals.
- VIP is a hormone that stimulates the secretion and inhibits the absorption of sodium, chloride, potassium, and water within the small intestine and increases bowel motility. These actions lead to a secretory diarrhea, hypokalemia, and dehydration, so-called Verner–Morrison syndrome.
- Imaging pattern with combination of cross-sectional imaging (CT and MRI), endoscopic ultrasound, and somatostatin receptor scintigraphy is similar to that of other neuroendocrine tumor of the pancreas (see Neuroendocrine tumor). VIPomas are typically solitary and greater than 3 cm in diameter with 75 % located in the tail of the pancreas. Sixty to 80 % are metastatic at the time of diagnosis, most commonly to the liver.

Suggested Reading

Batcher E, Madaj P, Gianoukakis AG (2011) Pancreatic neuroendocrine tumors. Endocr Res 36(1):35–43

Ha HK, Lee SH, Rha SE, Kim JH, Byun JY, Lim HK, Chung JW, Kim JG, Kim PN, Lee M-G, Auh YH (2000) Radiologic features of vasculitis involving the gastrointestinal tract. Radiographics 20:779–794

W

Waldenstrom Macroglobulinemia, GI Tract

- Waldenstrom macroglobulinemia is a low-grade lymphoid malignancy composed of mature plasmacytoid lymphocytes with production of abnormal monoclonal IgM protein. A macroglobulin proteinaceous hyaline material fills lacteals in lamina propria of the small bowel with lymphatic distension and edema.
- Mean age at diagnosis is 60 years old; symptoms are fatigue, weight loss, diarrhea, steatorrhea, malabsorption, and anemia. Most important for diagnosis is the IgM elevation with hyperviscosity syndrome (bleeding, visual changes, neurologic abnormalities).
- The small bowel is rarely involved with bowel dilatation and uniform diffuse thickening of valvulae conniventes.

Whipple Disease

- Whipple disease or intestinal lipodystrophy is a sporadically occurring chronic multisystem disease thought to be caused

P. Paolantonio, C. Dromain, *Imaging of Small Bowel, Colon and Rectum*,   173
A-Z Notes in Radiological Practice and Reporting,
DOI 10.1007/978-88-470-5489-9_23, © Springer-Verlag Italia 2014

by infection with an as yet unidentified Gram-positive bacterium (Tropheryma whipplei) closely related to actinobacteria.

- At histology glycoprotein from bacterial wall within foamy macrophages is present in the submucosa of the jejunum plus fat deposit within intestinal submucosa and lymph nodes causing lymphatic obstruction and leading to malabsorption.
- Symptoms are recurrent migratory arthralgias, malabsorption, abdominal pain, generalized peripheral lymphadenopathy, hyperpigmentation of the skin, and multiorgan involvement (liver, intestines, joints, heart, lung, CNS, eyes, and skin).
- At CT bulky (3–4 cm) large low-density (fatty content) lymph nodes in the mesenteric root and retroperitoneum, thickening of bowel wall, splenomegaly, ascites, pleuropericarditis, and sacroiliitis are detectable.
- Diagnosis is possible by means of endoscopically guided small bowel mucosa or peripheral lymph node biopsy. Differential diagnosis should consider sprue, amyloidosis, and lymphoma.
- Therapy is based on long-term broad-spectrum antibiotics.

Whirl Sign

- At computed tomography (CT), the appearance of the "whirl sign" is that of a soft tissue mass with an internal architecture of swirling strands of soft tissue and fat attenuation. The whirl sign is highly suggestive of intestinal volvulus that occurs when afferent and efferent bowel loops rotate around a fixed point of obstruction, which results in tightly twisted mesentery along the axis of rotation (for instance, closed loop bowel occlusion or sigmoid volvulus). These twisted loops of bowel and branching mesenteric vessels create swirling strands of soft tissue attenuation within a background of mesenteric fat attenuation, giving the appearance of a hurricane on a weather map.

Suggested Reading

Khurana B (2003) The whirl sign. Radiology 226:69–70

Waldenstrom J (1994) Incipient myelomatosis or "essential" hyperglobulin-
    emia with fibrinogenopenia-a new syndrome? Acta Med Scand
    117:216–247

Whipple GH (1907) A hitherto undescribed disease characterized anatomi-
    cally by deposits of fat and fatty acids in the intestinal and mesenteric
    lymphatic tissues. Bull Johns Hopkins Hosp 18:382–393

X

No lemma

P. Paolantonio, C. Dromain, *Imaging of Small Bowel, Colon and Rectum*,   177
A-Z Notes in Radiological Practice and Reporting,
DOI 10.1007/978-88-470-5489-9_24, © Springer-Verlag Italia 2014

Y

Yersinia enterocolitica

- *Yersinia enterocolitica* is a Gram-negative organism responsible of acute infective ulcerative enterocolitis. Symptoms are fever, diarrhea, and right lower quadrant pain. Infective diseases affect the terminal ileum and colon showing thickened folds plus ulceration, with lymphoid nodular hyperplasia. A differential diagnosis with acute appendicitis is not always possible based on clinical findings. However CT is useful to detect the normal appearance of the appendix identifying inflammatory changes of terminal ileum and cecum. A differential diagnosis based on imaging findings with Crohn's disease is not easy to perform. Some CT findings may indicate the lack of chronic inflammation of perivisceral fat (lack of fatty proliferation) and suggest an acute origin (marked perivisceral fat stranding) and thickening of cecal folds.
- Clinical features such as rapid onset of symptoms and quick recovery during antibiotic therapy are suggestive for infective enterocolitis. However stool culture analysis is essential in identifying the microorganism. If clinical or imaging findings still suggest a chronic inflammatory disease, patient management requires optical colonoscopy and biopsy.

P. Paolantonio, C. Dromain, *Imaging of Small Bowel, Colon and Rectum*, 179
A-Z Notes in Radiological Practice and Reporting,
DOI 10.1007/978-88-470-5489-9_25, © Springer-Verlag Italia 2014

Suggested Reading

Tuohy AMMM, O'Gorman M, Byington C, Barbara Reid W, Jackson D
(1999) Yersinia enterocolitis mimicking Crohn's disease in a toddler.
Pediatrics 104(3):36–41

Z

Zollinger–Ellison Syndrome

- Zollinger–Ellison syndrome is caused by a gastrinoma that is a non-beta islet cell gastrin-secreting tumor of the pancreas and/or the duodenum. Gastrin secretion stimulates the acid-secreting cells of the stomach to maximal activity, with consequent gastrointestinal mucosal ulceration. It may occur sporadically or as part of an autosomal dominant familial syndrome called multiple endocrine neoplasia type 1 (MEN 1).
- Clinical presentation associates a chronic diarrhea, heartburn, and severe recurrent ulcers of the esophagus, stomach, duodenum, and jejunum. The diagnosis of Zollinger–Ellison syndrome is made by raised blood levels of gastrin and the secretin stimulation test, which measures evoked gastrin levels. An increased level of chromogranin A is a common marker of neuroendocrine tumors.
- The primary tumor, the gastrinoma, is usually located in the pancreas and duodenum. Ectopic locations in the heart, ovary, and gallbladder have also been described. Gastrinomas may

occur as single tumors or as multiple, small tumors in particular if associated with a NEM1.

- The endo-ultrasonography is the imaging modality of choice for the detection of the tumor that is most often of small size. Moreover endoscopic-ultrasound allows to perform a tumor fine needle aspiration or biopsy.
- CT and MRI examinations require the acquisition of images during the late arterial phase (30 s after the initiation of contrast administration) as well as a portal venous phase and delayed phase. Tumors are either hypervascularized with early enhancement during the arterial phase or fibrous with more delayed enhancement.
- Gastrinomas are malignant in 60 % of cases. The most common sites of metastases are the liver and the abdominal lymph nodes. Somatostatin receptor imaging (using a scintigraphy or a PET technique) is indicated in combination with CT for the staging of the tumor.

Suggested Reading

Ito T, Cadiot G, Jensen RT (2012) Diagnosis of Zollinger-Ellison syndrome: increasingly difficult. World J Gastroenterol 18(39):5495–5503